THE IN-SYNC DIET

BY

GLYNIS BARBER

AND

FLEUR BORRELLI

Contents

About the Authors

Glynis Barber is a well-known British actress who has made a name for herself on stage and television. She is perhaps best known as Makepeace in the hugely successful worldwide hit TV series Dempsey and Makepeace. She has starred in numerous other TV series including Blake's 7, Night & Day, Emmerdale, The Royal and most recently Eastenders. She has also done a number of films and recently filmed the $100 million budget Hollywood remake of Point Break.

Glynis regularly appears on stage and her most recent production is the hit Broadway show, Beautiful (the Carole King story) at the Aldwych Theatre in the West End.

As well as acting, Glynis is also passionate about all aspects of health, nutrition and exercise. Recently she released her successful Yoga Secrets Anti-Ageing DVD (which quickly sold out on QVC) and she also launched her lifestyle/anti-ageing website:
www.AgelessbyGlynisBarber.com.
The website has proved very popular and continues to grow and expand.

Glynis trained at Mountview Theatre School.

Glynis is also on twitter @MsGlynisBarber

Fleur Borrelli PG Dip cPNI, BSc Nut Med, psycho-neuro-immunologist and nutritional therapist is one of the UK's first psycho-neuro-immunology clinicians. Psycho-neuro-immunology is a multi-layered approach to natural medicine, which looks at recovering the (biochemical, immunological, emotional, etc...) pathways to optimal health. It is based on the latest developments in the fields of psychology, neurology, endocrinology, immunology, evolutionary biology and epigenetics - all underpinned by nutritional medicine, exercise and psychosocial techniques.

Fleur is also a health writer and has appeared in many popular magazines and complementary healthcare journals. She is also a regular contributor to Glynis' Ageless website.

Fleur's website is www.NutritionandSuperfood.co.uk

Fleur can also be contacted by email Fleur@NutritionandSuperfood.co.uk and her clinic websites www.PutneyClinic.co.uk and www.BodiesUnderConstructionPhysio.com

Acknowledgements

I'd like to thank my lovely friend Gina To for the delicious recipes she came up with for the book. Gina writes a food blog, EatonSquareEdibles.com, where more of her her wonderful recipes can be found (but for the meantime, please ignore the naughty ones). I'd also like to thank Fleur for changing the way I eat and exercise and even how I drink water. I've never felt better.

Also my husband and son for putting up with my constant analysis of whatever they put in their mouths.

Thank you to Alex Segal at Cole Kitchenn and everyone at ROAR Global for helping to bring this book to fruition.

Glynis

My friend Nicki Edgell for creating the gluten-free baking recipes (see Chapter Fourteen) especially for The In-Sync Diet.

The Alliance for Natural Health International for their tireless campaigning to promote natural and sustainable approaches to healthcare worldwide.

Fleur

THE IN-SYNC DIET

Foreword by

Glynis Barber

Something strange happened to me in my twenties. From being a regular person who ate whatever she wanted without a second thought, I changed to a person completely passionate about what I was eating. Remaining healthy, free from illness, fit, youthful and being the best I can be at whatever age I am, has become integral to my life. It has led me to stray from my regular path of acting, to making an anti-aging Yoga DVD and starting a website dedicated to lifestyle and healthy ageing. I was inspired to do this by my genuine interest in the subject and as a response to the many times I get asked about how "I manage to stay so youthful".

So what exactly happened to me in my twenties? It was a surprisingly little thing, but demonstrates the power of a good teacher and how inspiration can have far reaching consequences.

I simply went to an aerobics class and the American instructor told us we had to jog as well as do her class and gave us books to read. "Get moving people!" she would yell at us, "Don't think just coming to this class is enough!" I had never read a book on nutrition or health and it had never occurred to me to do so. I don't even know why I listened to her, but I did and found a passion that has remained with me.

As the years have gone by and I have crept up in age, my interest in the subject knows no bounds. Suddenly all those diseases that seemed only for "old" people are beginning to happen to my peers. I am at "that age" where scary things can happen. No thank you very much. Not if I have anything to do about it. And that is where this book comes in.

Last summer, just as I was preparing to launch my website, I went to see nutritionist Fleur Borrelli. Little did I know that she would make changes to the way I eat and the way I exercise that would have a very profound effect on my life. I would lose inches, as well as just under a stone in weight. I would drop a dress size, gain lean muscle, have vastly improved energy levels, feel motivated and positive, all whilst eating a good amount of food.

The irony is that I went into all this very reluctantly. I didn't even go and see Fleur for this reason as I considered myself to be a very healthy eater, well educated in all aspects of nutrition. I went on the recommendation of an osteopath as I had quite a lot of unexplained joint pain. He suggested I go to find out if there was anything else going on other than simple mechanical injury. I wasn't keen. Don't nutritionists always start by telling you not to eat wheat? No matter what condition you have gone to see them for? The osteopath assured me that Fleur was very scientific and worked in an interesting way. So with a modicum of enthusiasm and a healthy dose of scepticism I went along. And surprise, surprise, she began to make changes to my diet immediately. Except that she was cunning. She saw my reluctance and broke me in slowly. And the process began. Slowly but surely I began to see big changes and found myself becoming a huge convert. Some of the ideas took a little getting used to because they were the opposite of what we've always been led to believe. However, when I committed to it fully, the results were fantastic.

This is the journey this book will offer you. We are talking about results to last a lifetime. We are talking about changes to how you will eat, drink and exercise forever. We are talking about the end of yo-yo dieting. But most importantly this book will empower you to take your health into your own hands...

Chapter One

Why we are all out-of-sync

At some point in your lives, most of you will have been on a diet. Some of you may well have spent a fortune on the many diet books, diet pills, diet services, meal replacements and other 'miracle cures' that there are on the market. But they haven't worked - why not? The reason is that you are still out-of-sync.

So let's look at the weight problem a little more closely. Since the 50's we have been getting bigger and bigger. Our bust size has increased by one and half inches, as have our hips. But worse still, our waists have increased by a whopping six and a half inches! And not only that, our mental and physical health is not that great either - anti-depressants are among the most commonly prescribed medications in modern medicine. And antacids are among the most commonly purchased over-the-counter products.

All your mental and physical health problems have a connection to a lack of energy and by this we mean chemical energy - otherwise known as adenosine tri-phosphate (ATP). Feeling constantly tired all the time represents one of the most common reasons why you visit your doctor. This is because up until 200 years ago your predecessors had a life that was much simpler than it is today. Certainly they were not bombarded with the constant demands for our attention that you are now. To cope with this relentlessness, you have to use 100% of your brain power rather than the 10% that people believe. This is an exhausting process.

You are surrounded by constant stress, food choices that your predecessors would never have dreamed of and very little opportunity to move around in the way your body needs. It is no wonder that you all have to watch your waistlines - food is available at every turn and you don't need to expend any energy to get it.

Did you know that your behaviour is regulated by daily rhythms known as circadian, or biorhythms? Circadian comes from the Latin 'circa' meaning around and diem meaning the daylight. This means the way you drink, the way you eat and the way you move are all very important for the way your body functions and the health of every organ in your body. To that end, you have thirteen clock genes all regulated by a master clock gene in the brain. Every organ in your body from your liver to your kidneys to your pancreas will be regulated by these clock genes.[1] Studies have shown that it is the disruption of these biorhythms that can contribute to conditions such as depression and seasonal affective disorder.[2] Your clock genes work best for you if you behave in the way you are designed for - eating when you are hungry, drinking when you are thirsty and sleeping when you are tired. But the tragedy is you don't even have the energy to act in this way anymore.

So now you are doing the reverse - you eat in case you get hungry. You have a cup of tea just to break up the day rather than drinking because we are thirsty. You don't sleep well because you don't have the energy to go to sleep and stay asleep. In terms of chemical energy, it is much more expensive to go to sleep than to stay awake. And then you resort to stimulants such as coffee when we get tired during the day, which can negatively affect your energy levels and drive up appetite.

And on top of this, because your brain uses the most energy of all the organs in your body, it really is the master controller of your metabolism.[1] The first signs of hunger appear because your brain needs some energy. Genetically you are programmed to move at this stage to go and hunt for food but what do you do instead? You eat! You do not rely on energy systems that there are in place to give you the boost you need to get going. Then you start trying to reduce the calories because you are then out-of-sync.

Nothing has been worse for your ability to maintain a good weight than the calorie-controlled diet. The calorie-controlled diet is based on the flawed assessment that if you eat foods with a low-calorie content you will be able to lose weight. Low-calorie foods can slow down your metabolism and stop you from losing weight because your brain senses there might be a calorie deficit. And, what is more, healthy foods with a higher calorie content may even keep your appetite at bay and stop you from overeating. And zero calorie drinks, for example, will increase your appetite and cause food cravings as you will discover later on.

When you are out-of-sync, you are more prone to weight gain, obesity, heart disease and a whole host of other health problems. So how do you survive this modern life, stay lean and healthy and full of vitality? **The In-Sync Diet** will show you how.

We felt compelled to write this book to share with you dietary and lifestyle tips on how to tone up and feel fantastic because you are *In-Sync*. We wrote it to empower you to be able to keep the weight off and continue to feel full of energy. We want to put an end to needless yo-yo dieting and feeling miserable about the way you look. We know we can help you to be *In-Sync.*

Footnotes

1.   Bunney W.E. and Bunney B.G. Molecular clock genes in man and
      lower animals: Possible implications for circadian abnormalities
      in depression. *Neuropsycopharmacology* (2000) 22, 835-845.

2.   Storch K.F and Lipan et al. Extensive and divergent circadian gene expression in liver and heart. *Nature* 417, 78-83; (2 May 2002).

3.   Peters A, Pellerin L et al. Causes of obesity: Looking beyond the hypothalamus. *Progress in Neurobiology,* Volume 81, Issue 2, Feb 2007, Pages 61-88.

Chapter Two

Why The In-Sync Diet works

Do you ever feel totally confused because all the advice you have been given seems to conflict? Do you eat three meals per day or do you eat six? Do you fast or do you never skip a meal? Do you have a low-fat diet or even a high protein diet?

Over the years, there have been a vast array of different diets and some have worked better than others but we can probably safely say that few have had any lasting effect:

The Low Fat Diet

Diets like the low-fat diet have actually made your expanding waistlines bigger and contributed to some of the major diseases in society today. Promoters of low-fat diets have encouraged you to eat high levels of carbohydrates on a regular basis. This has led to the dysregulation of blood sugar (glucose) control - a factor in most diseases.[1]

The Calorie-Controlled Diet

The calorie-controlled diet is based on the flawed assessment that if you eat foods with a low-calorie content you will be able to lose weight. The problem with this is that healthy foods with a higher calorie content may keep your appetite at bay and stop you from overeating. Low-calorie foods can slow down your metabolism and stop you from losing weight. And what is worse, zero calorie drinks will increase your appetite and cause food cravings as you discover later on.

The Low GI Diet

You are encouraged to eat a diet high in whole grains, for example, muesli, granola and cereal bars. As you will learn through The In-Sync Diet whole grains are not as healthy as they might seem. The low GI diet also promotes a low-fat diet, which as you have read is actually detrimental to health.

The Eating Little and Often Diet

Once fat was removed from your diet, you began to eat more carbohydrates, which really messed up your blood sugar levels. You became prone to dizzy spells and low energy if you did not eat. Advice then became 'eat little and often to stop those energy dips'. This well-intended advice has acted, in the same way that a sticking plaster has on a wound - it temporarily stops the problem, but it is not the solution.

The Plant-based Diet

This method of dieting relies on eating vegetables, grains, legumes and fruit with little or no animal foods. As you will learn about the foods to eat on The In-Sync Diet, you will understand how the consumption of grains and legumes can damage your health by causing inflammation.[2] We are not talking inflammation that occurs when you have an injury that occurs in a particular part of the body. We are talking about inflammation that can start off in the gut and can spread through the whole body. This general inflammatory state that we can get ourselves into is made worse by stress. When we are inflamed, we are unable to lose weight. Consequently, we are susceptible to inflammation and obesity.[3]

The Fast a little then eat what you like Diet

In the West, fasting is currently being used successfully as a means to weight loss. Unlike some nations, we in the West do not really enjoy restricting our calories and so fasting is a new way for us to try to reduce our waistlines but positively impact our health as well. But are we doing it right? Done in the right way it can be an incredibly effective way of shifting fat. But done in the wrong way we may be at risk of losing healthy muscle tissue. And certainly what we should not be doing after putting our bodies through a period of cleanse is to then bombard it with all the wrong kinds of foods that will overload your digestive system and undo all the good work that you have done.

In-Sync will provide you with a common sense, easy-to-follow programme that will help you to burn fat, feel more energised than ever before and increase your longevity. *In-Sync* is the new generation of diet that will turn everything you have been told on its head....

So let's start right away by busting a few common myths that there are out there that are affecting our ability to be **In-Sync**.

Myth Busted: Grains, especially whole-grains are healthy and non-fattening

On the whole, grains and cereals have only been consumed in large amounts in the diet for the last 10,000 years, since the Agricultural Revolution. We began to cultivate crops to avoid starvation but in the last 10,000 year's research has shown that our brain is decreasing in size, we are losing muscle mass and becoming fatter. What is going on? Well, the fact is that processed refined grain products such as white bread, pasta and other bakery goods typically have no natural fibre and contain bleaching agents, synthetic vitamins and artificial colourings. They have the potential to do us harm by disturbing our blood sugar levels and adding to our toxic load which we will talk about in chapter four. This has led to a move back towards what has been thought of as a much healthier option - whole grains. Whole grains are exactly as the name suggests   grains that remain intact. They have not had their outer coating removed and are thought to be more nutritious, non-fattening and, for this reason, more healthy. But this may not be the case because whole grains gather moulds which are very difficult to remove and can cause inflammation.[1] Whole grains also contain chemicals that can damage your gut and cause inflammation. These chemicals can also impact on your ability to lose weight.[4]

Myth Busted: Eating fat makes you fat and damages your health

Diets like the low-fat diet have actually made our expanding waistlines bigger and contributed to some of the major diseases in society today. Promoters of low-fat diets have encouraged us to eat high levels of carbohydrates on a regular basis. This has led to the dysregulation of blood sugar (glucose) control - a factor in most diseases.[1] Contrary to popular belief, eating moderate amounts of healthy fat do not get stored as fat. We know that olive oil, for example, gets used in cell membranes and that the largest amount of cholesterol in the body can be found in the brain. Moderate fat intake is also vitally important for your mental function and, in fact, the function of every cell of every tissue in your body. Without it, you will more readily succumb to food cravings, increased appetite and health problems.

On the other hand, relying too heavily on carbohydrates such as bread, cakes, pasta or pastries will definitely make you put on weight because they get converted to the fat that sits around your waistline.

Eating healthy fat has even more advantages. It can keep you feeling fuller for longer and help to stop the cravings. **The In-Sync Diet** will help you to include healthy fats that are vital for great looking hair and skin and to improve your mood.

Myth Busted: Eating lots of red meat should be part of a weight loss diet

High amounts of meat have been encouraged by a number of weight loss diets in the last few decades. It is based on the correct assumption that by increasing protein and reducing grains you will burn fat. This is reportedly how our Stone Age ancestors would have eaten but certainly not on a daily basis. We know from findings of bones in caves that they would have relied principally on eating fish, seafood and birds. They would have stocked up occasionally with red meat when they were able to make a big kill.

The problem is that meat reared nowadays is very different from that which your ancestors would have eaten. They would have eaten meat from animals that had had proper exercise. Produce from animals that have had very little exercise and have been grain-fed contain too high a proportion of unhealthy fats and too low a proportion of protein. Red meat consumption has therefore been linked to autoimmune disease, cardiovascular disease, cancer and other health conditions.[5] Grass-fed organic meat, on the other hand, tends to be higher in the healthy fat omega-3 and is a healthy option.

Eating *moderate* amounts of good sources of protein is very important in **The In-Sync Diet**, particularly eggs, fish meat and nuts. For those that do eat animal protein, the more the animal has exercised, the better. Our bodies do not store protein so we need to eat sufficient amounts each day.

Myth Busted: Water should be sipped through the day to keep you hydrated

We have been encouraged since the rise of the sports drink industry in the 80's to keep ahead of thirst and drink continually and often. The problem with drinking little and often is that instead of being well hydrated, we actually become dehydrated. This is because we never drink enough at one time for our cells to really amass sufficient liquid. We also lose the sense of thirst with these constant mini top-ups. We lose the sense of whether we are actually thirsty and can trick ourselves into thinking that we are hungry instead and we get food cravings. So becoming dehydrated can actually make us fat. When our cells become dehydrated, they go into survival mode and store fat as this will provide us with energy in an emergency situation. For every litre of water our body loses, we compensate with a kilo of fat! Find out in the next chapter of **The In-Sync Diet** exactly how you can overcome this.

Myth Busted: Breakfast is the most important meal of the day and will stop you from overeating

Breakfast has always been touted as the most important meal of the day. By eating breakfast, we are told we are avoiding unnecessary blood sugar dips and are less likely to overeat later on. Wrong. What is interesting is that breakfast coincides with our cortisol circadian peak. Cortisol is an activity hormone, necessary to get us going in the morning. Its job is to promote the release of sugar into the bloodstream so that we have enough energy to move. We really don't need food at this point, our body is taking care of the problem all by itself. The problem with eating breakfast at this time, before we even feel hungry, is that double the amount of sugar goes into the bloodstream. Because having too much sugar running around the bloodstream is bad for us, the body packs everything away far too quickly and the net effect is that we soon feel hungry again. This can be made worse by the fact that our breakfast choices are often processed sugary cereals. We are out-of-sync. **The In-Sync Diet** will transform the way you think about breakfast.

Myth Busted: We should eat 'little and often'

Genetically we are not designed for frequent meal intake. It is a response to the problems associated with our contemporary society - low blood sugar. Because our blood sugar levels are unstable, we rely on having to eat constant snacks throughout the day. But we can train our body to behave in the way it should, and in doing so the weight will fall off. You will learn that it really is okay to feel hungry and that it's *healthy* because it gives you a signal to move and find food. And moving to find food helps regulate our metabolism and gives our brain the right signal so we can lose weight. We have a large gland called the pancreas, which really has to do an awful lot of work. Every time we eat, it has to produce digestive enzymes to help us digest our food. This uses up an awful lot of chemical energy (Adenosine Tri-Phosphate), which could be better off spent elsewhere. We also know that the pancreas needs to repair itself between meals and so snacking will put unnecessary strain on an organ that ultimately plays a crucial role.[6]

Myth Busted: Fasting can be done on a regular basis without exercise

The tradition of fasting is centuries old. Currently, this ancient tradition is being revived because of its beneficial impact on the body weight. Fasting can help to burn fat, stabilise blood sugar levels and improve our vitality. And we definitely are still genetically programmed to be able to suffer periods of famine but only under certain conditions. This type of fast/feast way of behaving really sorts our genes out so that they switch on and off when they should. And the more they do this, the better our metabolism works. If you move about before you eat, your body has systems in place to be much more efficient at getting its fuel. We will tell you more about this in Chapter Seven, but suffice to say that it is the time in between meals when your body has no other option, but to burn fat. Successful fasting depends on a healthy metabolism that will allow your energy system to kick into fat burn once all the stored energy in your body runs out. This may not happen straight away on a weight loss programme because your body is not used to using fat as an energy source, it tends to prefer sugar or glucose instead. And the danger of this is that instead of burning the fat, you may break down healthy lean tissue. This may look good on the scales but will predispose you to weight gain once you are off the programme. The *In-Sync* programme will take you carefully through the steps to successfully introduce healthy fasting into your life and burn fat not lean tissue while being in a fasting state.

So you see that to be **In-Sync** you need to get the balance right between not only what you are eating, but also the way you are doing it.

The In-Sync Diet

The In-Sync Diet will take you to new levels of weight management and appetite control. We will show you how you can burn fat even when you are not eating. And you will not be hungry because you will not be denied food. You will also be able to eat like a king! Unlike current fasting diets, we will ensure that you also become more efficient at storing energy when you eat, in such a way that you will not put on weight after the programme. Your body will become so energy-efficient that you will no longer suffer the constant pangs of hunger or food cravings. We will liberate you from having to think about food all day. You will have the mental clarity and focus you have always wanted to have. And unlike calorie restricted/fasting diets, you will not lose muscle which means you will continue to burn fat, should you wish, way beyond our programme.

Why Diets Fail?	The In-Sync Solution
Get hungry	You will become so energy efficient that hunger will be a thing of the past
Can't ignore the food cravings	You will become so energy efficient that food cravings will disappear
All calories are equal	Your programme will include calorie dense foods that will sustain your energy levels
Low in fat	Your programme will include a moderate amount of fat to keep you healthy and not hungry
Calories are restricted	You will be able to feast like a king!
Reliant on eating little and often	Thinking about your next snack will be a thing of the past
Having to constantly think about what you are eating	You will not be made to go out and buy foods that cannot be easily found in the supermarket
Dizziness and headaches	You will burn fat even when you are not eating to provide energy - a lack of which is often the cause of dizziness and headaches
Unpleasant digestive symptoms	You will not be eating foods that wreak havoc with your digestion
Low mood	Your brain will not be denied energy
Feelings of denial	When you eat, you can feast
Too much red meat	You will be shown a number of healthy proteins
Loss of muscle tissue when fasting	Fasting will be correctly applied so you are not wasting healthy muscle tissue
Dehydration	Hydration is an important part of the programme

What you can expect to do on the In-Sync:

The In-Sync Diet will last just eight weeks. By the end of eight weeks, you will be surprised at how your body shape has changed and your cravings are gone.

- Eat the foods that will help you to lose weight not hinder you.
- Most of what you need to buy will be easily available in a supermarket.
- Eat sufficient amounts of healthy protein to increase your muscle tone.
- Enjoy a high amount of vegetables cooked in delicious ways as a healthy carbohydrate source.
- Cut out gluten and cereal grains that can damage your waistline and your gut and negatively affect your brain chemistry.
- Try different durations of fasting in such a way that you will effectively fat burn without losing healthy muscle tissue.
- Eat healthy fat that will not only help you burn fat, it will also improve your mood.
- Introduce exercise into your daily routine in ways you did not know possible.

What you can expect to learn on the In-Sync:

- You will learn how to become energy efficient. By being more energy efficient, you will be able to go for longer periods without food. The cells that make up your tissues and organs will become better at getting the fuel they need without you even needing to eat more than you should. By being more efficient at storing energy as well as using energy, you will be leaner than you have ever been before. You will also be much healthier. Lack of energy efficiency can be associated with most chronic diseases including neurological diseases.
- You will be eating a diet that is delicious and satisfying and rich in nutrients. This will ensure that you get above and beyond your daily intake of vitamins and minerals.
- You will discover how instead of being fattening and damaging to our health, certain fats will actually help you to lose weight, have better hormonal control and you will notice how much your hair and skin quality improves.
- You will find out how by being in tune with the whole of your body, you can maintain a healthy metabolism that will help to keep the fat off way beyond our programme. You will learn how to be *In-Sync.*

Fleur - Case Study

I had a client who came to me for a number of reasons including weight loss. She had also been suffering from recurring infections for a number of years that she could not shake off. She successfully managed to give up smoking three years prior to coming to our consultation and that was when the weight started to pile on. Her blood sugar levels were so unstable that she did not dare leave the house without eating first and was packing a number of snacks to get her through until lunchtime. She was eating six meals per day and these were mostly grain based. She would get terrible migraines if she did not eat. She had lost touch with what her body needed to be lean, healthy and strong. She was completely confused as to what dietary advice she should follow. She was out-of-sync. She was given the *In-Sync* programme to follow and her infections cleared up. The pounds fell off her and she regained her natural biorhythm that prevented her from having constant cravings and being dependent on constant snacking to keep her energy levels stable. Find out how...

Footnotes

1. E.S. Ford. Risks for all-cause mortality, cardiovascular disease and diabetes associated with the metabolic syndrome. *Diabetes Care* Volume 28, No 7, pp 1769-1778. July 2005.

2. Muskiet FAJ. The evolutionary background, cause and consequences of chronic systemic low-grade inflammation. Significance for clinical chemistry. *Ned Tijdschr Klin ChemcLabgeneesk,* 36:199-214. 2011.

3. Serhan C.N. Resolution phase of inflammation: novel endogenous anti-inflammatory and proresolving lipid mediators and pathways. *Annu Rev Immunol* 2007, 25:101-137 2007

4. Cordain L. www.meandmydiabetes.com/2011/12/03/loren-cordain-leaky-gut-whole-grain-and-even-potatoes. December 3, 2011

5. Oliver J.E, and Silman A.J. Risk factors for the development of rheumatoid arthritis. *Scandanavian Journal of Rheumatology.* 2006, vol 35, No 3, pages 169-174.

6. Pruimboom L. Pancreatic enzymes the missing link in health and disease. *European Association of Clinical Psycho-neuro-immunology.* 2014.

Chapter Three

Getting back your thirst - Why it is important

We mentioned in Chapter One the importance of good health and maintaining a toned physique of living in accordance with our circadian rhythms. We can look to evolution for more clues as to why this came about. The hypothesis is we call migrated out of Africa around 60,000 years ago.[1] Our survival in Africa depended on us being able to hunt for food when all the lions and other predators were asleep. This meant us having to develop a 'active during the day/asleep at night' rhythm that our genetic make-up is geared towards and our body functioning depends on. And this goes for the way we drink - we should use our inherent ability to drink according to the dictates of thirst. And yet we have become a 'water obsessed' nation to the point that it is our conscience if we do not carry that bottle of water around with us or have it on our desk. And then there is *that* '8 X 8' rule that tells us to have eight eight ounce glasses of water throughout the day. So why are we following it?

Hydration and sporting performance

Before the 80's the only recommendations that were given regarding hydration were to drink according to thirst. This is something that children do very well instinctively. Nowadays we are encouraged to stay ahead of thirst as if mild dehydration was a disease, which it certainly isn't. The sports drinks industry has much to blame for this and it has been very much in their favour to promote the idea that performance may be enhanced by the constant intake of fluids to 'drink to stay ahead of thirst'. This is merely a hypothesis that has not been supported by scientific evidence.[2] What has been forgotten in recent decades is that if you allow your thirst to dictate, you will be alerted by a special sensing system in your brain that you need to consume water when you are merely two percent dehydrated. Really thirst is all about regulating the thickness or osmolality of the blood.[3] If your brain detects your blood is getting too thick, it will drive up thirst so that you will drink and your blood will become thinner again. Conversely, if your blood is thin enough, then you will not be thirsty. Our body's natural inclination is to naturally 'osmoregulate' and so if we drink too little then water can be drawn from the bones and this can cause bone issues later on.[4] It is all about keeping a balance and you will do this naturally if you are *In-Sync*.

We have become chronic tea and coffee drinkers

The problem is that we tend to drink 'chronically' throughout the day. Tea drinking was once an afternoon ritual to bridge the gap between lunchtime and dinner but nowadays it occurs as a means to divide the working day into well-earned breaks. The problem with this is that your poor old brain does not understand this social custom and gets concerned that you are losing too much fluid. Too much fluid loss means too much sodium loss. This means the body will have to do what it can to retain it, such as drive up blood pressure [3] or give us puffy feet and ankles because of oedema. [5]

The continual intake of liquid through the day is making us fat

Our cells then respond by going into survival mode and when they are in survival mode they throw out water and retain FAT. Yes, that is correct. *The continual drinking of inconsequential amounts of liquid throughout the day can really make you fat!* This is because our cells have a special plumbing system that will either transport water, glucose or fat into the cells depending on our metabolic needs at the time. [6] If we are drinking out-of-

28

sync e.g. constantly through the day but not sufficient at one single time, then we will store fat. Fat acts as the body's emergency storage tank to be burnt for energy in times of need. And when this happens, it is because your brain thinks you are in need of some help. When the cells lose water they tend to store fat.

Avoiding water intoxication and chronic dehydration

That does not mean that you should go out and drink more and more water because 'water intoxication' is very dangerous. And as we have said earlier, sensible advice seems to be to 'drink according to thirst' rather than 'drink to stay ahead of thirst.' Instead, think back to how you used to behave as a child. You would probably run around and be active until the need to have a drink took over. And so you had to stop what you were doing and satiate your thirst before you could carry on your game. Your brain will naturally stop the 'thirsty feeling' at a certain point when you are around 80% hydrated to avoid the danger of drinking too much. This is a completely natural way of behaving and gives your cells the perfect opportunity to fill up their water tanks. And in this way, your brain will not start to employ emergency measures and your cells will not store fat.

Chronic dehydration, instead of being a moment in time, can build up slowly over the years until your weight and your health begins to suffer. The problem with thirst is that if you do not satiate it at that moment, you may lose the thirsty feeling and begin to crave food instead or it can even manifest as pain.[7]

Whilst it is not possible to give a standard answer as to how much you need to drink, **The In-Sync Diet** would like to give you a few guidelines. We feel it is important to get this right before you start the programme:

- Drink approximately 35mls water for every kilo of body weight.
- Drink plenty of water when you first wake up as your body will have been in a 'fasting' state overnight.
- This should be at least a pint of water or maybe two depending on your body size.
- You may then follow this with your usual mug of tea or coffee if that is what you like to have.
- Then do not drink again until you are thirsty.
- There will be times when you need to drink more such as after playing sport or before and after a sauna.
- Those who are susceptible to kidney stones should also be very careful to make sure that you do not go far beyond the 2% dehydration.

- Fluid intake may need to be higher when drinking alcohol.

Top Tip: If your urine is a pale straw colour you have a good indication that you are drinking enough liquid.

Can drinks with artificial sweeteners replace water?

In clinic, when I measure my clients to see their improvement I always make sure that their total body water has not gone down. Some clients do not like drinking water because they find it boring or they don't like the taste of it. This is fine as long as they find a replacement that does not have any sugar or artificial sweeteners in it. The problem with sweetened drinks is of course that they contain sugar and sugar has calories, which may prevent you from reaching your target weight loss goal. And there is another problem... Your brain does not perceive sugary drinks as a liquid but as a food, which may get the fat storage tanks going again.[8] Why not go for one of the many different sugar-free herbal teas that there are in the supermarket instead or even green tea, which may even help with burning fat? The very latest research shows that sugar substitutes such as saccharin can affect weight gain and obesity by the way they influence bacteria in the human gut.[9]

What about artificially sweetened drinks?

Artificial sweeteners will wreak havoc with your metabolism and make you completely out-of-sync. While it is correct that they do not contain calories it is not true that you will not put on weight by drinking them. Your brain cannot be tricked for long. It is very efficient at detecting the number of calories a food has. One of the problems with artificial sweeteners is that they can be up to two hundred times sweeter than sugar to the taste, without the calories. Your brain expects these calories from the sweeteners and then realises that it has not been given them. It, therefore, increases your appetite to get what it expected.[10] So in order to shift the pounds, you should stick to drinking either plain old water or herbal replacements as and when you need to; not because you feel you should, or you have just met up with a friend and want to mark the social occasion with a huge latte.

Is coffee okay to drink on the *In-Sync* Programme?

Coffee contains caffeine which has a stimulatory effect on your nervous system. It is often used as a means to stay awake (although water would be a better option). It is also fairly addictive when drunk in quantity causing withdrawal symptoms such as headaches, nausea, muscle fatigue and irritability. Past research has demonstrated that it can reduce the absorption of a number of vitamins and minerals in particular vitamin C and calcium.[11] It has been linked with a number of health problems including anxiety, insomnia, osteoporosis and peptic ulcers.

However, despite all the negatives it is now receiving some better press. It contains compounds which may actually support your antioxidant systems reducing the likelihood of reduced cognitive functioning in older age.[12]

So, drunk in moderation, coffee may have some beneficial effects. It has been included in the *In-Sync* programme but only with meals. It is best to choose an organic variety to avoid the pesticides and fertilisers that the leaves are heavily sprayed with. If possible, invest in a grinder and grind your own beans. In this way, you will enjoy the richer, fuller flavour while still maintaining the antioxidants and minerals from the beans. Avoid instant coffee at all costs, which contains high amounts of acrylamide - a known carcinogen.[13] Add a spoonful of coconut oil to your freshly brewed coffee to give you a boost of energy and a pinch of cinnamon for extra flavour.

Is it better to drink coconut water instead of normal water?

Coconut water, a product that has fairly recently flooded the market, comes from young green coconuts that are harvested when the flesh inside is soft and rubbery. In tropical countries such as Brazil, it has been served on beaches in its natural form for years. Nowadays it is packaged up and consumed worldwide - its popularity soaring because of its natural isotonic properties. According to The American Journal of Emergency Medicine, it has an electrolyte composition that is perfect to be used intravenously in remote parts of the globe where there may not be saline solution available.[14] Sports people are, for this reason, choosing it over their more artificial electrolyte sports energy drinks. Its natural sugars provide energy and it is bursting with vitamins and minerals including calcium, potassium, magnesium and zinc.

Use it for braising meat; it adds a wonderful subtle flavour. *Be aware, however, that it does contain calories due to the fairly high sugar content, which comprises of around seventy-five percent glucose and twenty-five percent fructose. It should never be considered a water replacement.*

So by establishing these basic fundamentals regarding hydration you are already well on the road to successfully reaching your weight loss goals. By putting into practice your 'bulk drinking' instead of the constant fluid intake all through the day you will begin to be *In-Sync*. And when you are *In-Sync* your metabolism works so much better and you will begin to burn the fat. And you may even find that instead of being hungry you had been thirsty all along!

Footnotes

1.   Tattrsall I. Human Origins: Out of Africa.
      www.pnas.org/content/106/38/16018.full
2.   Noakes T.D. Is drinking to thirst optimum. *Annals of Nutrition & Metabolism.* Vol 57. Suppl. 2, 2010.
3.   McDonough A.A. Mechanisms of proximal tubule sodium transport regulation that link extracellular fluid volume and blood pressure. *American Journal of Physiolog.* Vol 298, No 1, R851-856. 1 April 2010.
4.   Adams, M.A. What is intervertebral disc degeneration and what causes it? *Spine.* Vol. 31, Issue 18, pp 2151-2161. 15 August 2006.

5. Keefer A. Does sodium and potassium imbalance lead to swollen ankles. http://www.livestrong.com/article/520918-sodium-and-potassium-imbalance-and-swelling-ankles/

6. Agre P. The aquaporin water channels. *Proc. Am. Thorac. Soc.* 3(1): 5-13. 2006.

7. Ogino Y., Kakeda T. et al. Dehydration enhances pain-evoked activation in the human brain compared with rehydration. *Anaesthesia & Analgesia.* Vol. 118, Issue 6, pp 1317-1325. June 2014.

8. Rippe J.M. and Saltzman E. Sweetened beverages and health. Current state of scientific understanding. *Advances in Nutrition.* Vol 4, pp527-529. September 2013.

9. Suez J. et al. Artificial Sweeteners induce glucose intolerance by altering the gut microbiota. *Nature,* doi:10.1038/nature13793, 17th September 2014.

10. Rudenga K.L., Small D.M. Amygdulla response to sucrose consumption is inversely related to artificial sweetener use. *Appetite.* Vol 58, Issue 2, pages 504-507. April 2012

11. Barger-Lux M.J., Heaney R.P. and Stegman M.R. Effects of moderate caffeine intake on the calcium economy of premenopausal women. Am J. Clin. Nutr. Vol 52 no 4 pp722-725, October 1990.

12. Abreu R.V., Silva-Oliveira E.M. et al. Chronic coffee and caffeine ingestion effects on the cognitive function and antioxidant system of rat brains. *Pharmacology, Biochemistry and Behaviour.* Vol. 91, issue 4, pp659-664. 4 October 2011.

13. Larsson S., Akesson A. and Wolk A. Dietary acrylamide intake and prostate cancer risk in prospective cohort of Swedish men. *Cancer Epidemiology Biomarkers& Prevention.* 18, 139. June 2009.

14. Campbell-Falck, Thomas T. et al. The intravenous use of coconut water. *The American Journal of Emergency Medicine.* Vol 18, issue 1, pp 108-111. January 2000.

Chapter Four

An overview of The In-Sync Diet

The In-Sync Diet will take you through the five distinct phases of our programme which lasts eight weeks. As you progress through, you will learn how to burn fat, tone up and generally feel better all over. In weeks one and two you will be eating three healthy and delicious meals per day. During weeks three and four you will be learning the secrets of healthy fasting to ditch the fat, not lean tissue. But unlike other diets, you will not have to restrict calories on those days. You will still be able to eat well without putting the weight back on. By weeks five and six you will be on a roll, you will have lost your cravings and your energy dips and you will be looking and feeling fantastic. During weeks seven and eight your body will be shedding the pounds and you will not even feel hungry.

Getting back your thirst - Why it is important

The In-Sync Diet Phase One - Two-Day Preparation
Two-day gut 'clear-out'

- Measuring yourself
- Gently shifting the toxins
- The two-day cleanse

The In-Sync Diet Phase Two - Weeks One and Two
Three enjoyable meals per day with five-hour gaps in between

- Healthy foods to reduce your lectin load beyond gluten
- Regulating blood sugar levels by moving away from eating 'little and often'

Getting Moving Chapter - Becoming a fat burner, not a sugar burner

The In-Sync Diet Phase Three - Weeks Three and Four

- Why breakfast isn't necessarily the best option
- Getting enough sleep to maintain your circadian rhythm

Getting Moving Chapter - The long and slow workout

The In-Sync Diet Phase Four - Weeks Five and Six

Eating well on two meals per day

- Top twelve superfoods to repair your mitochondria
- Stress and healthy hormone balance

Getting Moving Chapter:

Part One: Training your large muscle groups

Part Two: Yoga for stress relief

The In-Sync Diet Final Phase - Weeks Seven and Eight

- The luxury meal - eating your brain happy
- Lose weight by burning fat for heat regulation

Getting Moving Chapter - Moving in everyday life

The In-Sync Diet Maintenance

Have you tried every diet under the sun and nothing has worked? Are you fed up with constant calorie counting and denying yourself foods? Are you spending whole days fasting and still not losing weight? Do you feel you are not being given enough choices? Want to reach your fat burning potential? **The In-Sync Diet** is for you.

Measuring yourself - are weight scales the right way to go?

Now you have got hydration right you are almost ready to go! The next thing you may want to think about is how to monitor your weight throughout the programme. I tend to tell every client that comes to see me for weight loss not to look at the scales in case the act of doing so throws them out-of-sync! This is because everyday bathroom scales are not able to tell you what is going on in your body very accurately. They won't inform you about how well you are doing on the *In-Sync.* You won't know whether you are burning fat, which is what you want.

Be assured the hydration part of this diet is crucial. I used to be one of those who went through the day clutching a bottle of water and continually taking sips terrified of being dehydrated. Isn't it odd how scared we all are of that? It took a while to get my head around the fact that drinking like this can make you fat (see chapter 3) and paradoxically can also make you dehydrated. However, I have now seen the evidence of how drinking in bulk only when thirsty can make a huge difference to your weight.

Scales that tell you more

One of the ways you can monitor your hydration is by buying yourself a good set of scales that are able to measure what is known as **Total Body Water**. It is important for sustained fat burn that your total body water should gradually go up to between 50 - 60% or higher if you are an athlete. This is all about learning to drink, as you would have done naturally as a child, as we outlined in Chapter Three. You really should allow yourself to get a little thirsty and then drink enough to feel satiated. This could be one or two pints of water depending on your body size. We have recommended 35mls for every kilo of body weight as a rule of thumb.

If you really feel you need to measure your progress by

the scales, make sure you have scales that give you more information than just what you weigh. A good set of scales should also be able to tell you your **body fat** percentage as compared with your **lean tissue or muscle mass** percentage. It is lean tissue that will give you that beautiful toned appearance. The more **lean tissue/ muscle mass** you have, the more fat you will burn. You will become a fat burner, not a sugar burner.

Set the intention to weigh yourself only occasionally rather than every day. Or not at all should you wish - you will be able to tell by how well your clothes are fitting you. What might be useful for you is to measure yourself at the end of each phase of the programme just to keep motivated by how well your body is responding.

Glynis' Tip:

If there is any way you can get the scales that Fleur recommends, it's well worth it. I was fortunate enough to have Fleur do all my measuring and it was incredibly instructive. However, do not get obsessed with the scales. I personally would only weigh myself once a week at most. The idea is to lose fat and at the same time gain lean muscle (oh yes, you're going to have to get moving on this diet). Muscle is heavier than fat so a normal scale is not going to show you the true result. You may think you're not losing weight or are even gaining weight. At the very least you can use a tape measure...or just look in the mirror. You should also feel a difference in how your clothes fit.

Hip To Waist Measurement

If you do not want to buy a new set of scales, there are plenty of other ways you can measure yourself. You could get your tape measure out. Put it around the narrowest part of your waist above your hips. Make a note of the width but make sure you are not holding your stomach in! Then do the same around your hips at the widest part of the buttocks. Then get your calculator out and divide your waist circumference by your hip circumference and compare your results with the table below.

Females	Estimated health Risk	Estimated Body Shape
0.80 or below	Low	Pear
0.81 to 0.85	Moderate	Avocado
0.85+	High	Apple
Males	Estimated health Risk	Estimated Body Shape
0.95 or below	Low	Pear
0.96 to 1.0	Moderate	Avocado
1.0+	High	Apple

Chapter Five

Phase One of The In-Sync Diet

Gently shifting the toxins

It has been estimated that humans have found, created or used five million chemicals in all, mainly in the last few decades.[1] Mostly we are talking xenobiotics, foreign chemicals that we come into contact with when we eat, when we breathe and those we absorb through our skin. There are now seventy-five thousand chemicals in everyday use.[2] Our body also produces its own toxins as part of our normal metabolism.

Fortunately, we have evolved a complex network of systems to get rid of toxins that have been created internally. The antioxidant system cleverly destroys free radicals during chemical reactions in our cells before they can damage the cell itself. The liver is there to ensure that toxins are excreted out of the body in urine via the kidneys. Sweating can lose any heavy metals lurking about, not to mention the shedding of toxins via skin, hair and nails.

This is what happens when all is working well... But we now live in a modern environment where we are being overloaded with toxins. We have plastics in our toothpaste, herbicides in the air we breathe, synthetic hormones in our drinking water, heavy metals in our deodorant, harmful electromagnetic radiation in our homes, additives in our foods, the list goes on. Scientists estimate that everyone alive today carries within her or his body at least 700 contaminants, most of which have not been well studied.[3]

We may reach a point in our evolution where we have adapted to this environment of chemicals that are foreign to our body, but we haven't got there yet. We are succumbing more and more to symptoms produced by compromised detoxification systems such as poor digestion, headaches, depression and chronic fatigue.

The In-Sync Diet is going to take you through a very gentle cleanse to start to shift some of those chemicals that may get stuck in your fatty tissue and stop you from looking or feeling as good as you could. We do **not** recommend extreme dieting or juice fasts which can often make people feel much worse than they did before.

Taking out 'new' foods

75% of the foods you are eating now are 'new foods'. 'New foods' are foods that we are not genetically designed to be eating such as processed foods. Because we are not equipped to deal with these new foods, they tend not to get digested very well. If you have eaten processed or convenience foods, sugary foods and sandwiches on a daily basis, this cleanse is definitely for you. It will sort your gut out completely! And, what's more, your good bacteria in the gut will love it. And the more they love it, the better your metabolism will become.[4] And the better your metabolism becomes, the more fat you will lose and the less beholden you will be to your appetite. You will be *In-Sync*!

The Two-Day Gentle Clear-Out

Breakfast: ½ kilo steamed/raw veg (includes salad)

Lunch: ½ kilo steamed/raw veg (includes salad)

Dinner: ½ kilo steamed/raw veg (includes salad)

Top Tips:

- 2 teaspoons of apple cider vinegar per day over your vegetables. Apple cider vinegar has been linked to increased weight loss as well as a reduction in waist circumference and abdominal fat.[5]
- Avocado can be used as an 'oil' source during these two days - choose one that is sufficiently ripe and spread it over your vegetables or salad.
- If you digestion is compromised at all i.e. you suffer from abdominal discomfort it is better to cook your vegetables rather than to eat them raw.

Glynis' Tip:

I have to be honest, this two-day cleanse was the worst part of the entire process for me. But it's really important to cleanse out your system before starting the diet.

Eating only steamed vegetables can be really hard. Having a small portion of steamed veggies on the side of a meal is one thing, but a huge plate of the stuff I found very unappealing. It's what I did on the first day and, to be honest, I would have preferred not to eat at all. If, like me, you find this hard, then replace with raw vegetables. There is nothing wrong with munching on some raw carrots, tomatoes, radishes, celery, etc. However, do add some nice steamed greens.

I would suggest doing this on a weekend when you don't have much to do and you can relax. Obviously going out for a meal or a drink is not an option so best to lay low for these 2 days. And remember...it's only 2 days!! The rest of the diet is easy peasy compared to this.

Vegetables to choose from

Non-root vegetables

Artichokes	Greens: pak choy, Swiss chard, kale, spinach, mustard, beet greens
Asparagus	
Aubergine	Lettuce/mixed greens: romaine, red and green leaf, endive, spinach, rocket, radicchio, watercress, chicory
Bamboo shoots	
Bean sprouts	
Bell or other peppers	Mange tout
Broccoli	Mushrooms
Brussels sprouts	Okra
Cabbage (all types)	Radishes
Cauliflower	Salsa (sugar-free)
Celery	Sea vegetables (kelp, etc.)
Courgettes	Sugar snap peas
Chives, onion, leeks, garlic	Tomatoes/mixed vegetable juice
Cucumber	
Green Beans	Water chestnuts

Root-vegetables or high starch vegetables

These are high in energy they will be limited in Chapter Six.

Beetroot	Pumpkin
Butternut squash	Swede
Carrots	Sweet potato
Parsnip	Turnip
Mandioca	Celeriac
Plantain	Tapioca

Getting your five-a-day

It has been officially reaffirmed again that eating just five daily portions of fruit and vegetables is associated with a lower risk of death from any cause.[6] Food rich in plant chemicals, known as 'phytonutrients', and antioxidants will have tremendous benefits for good health and longevity.

And yet new research published in the *British Journal of Nutrition* says there is an alarming shortfall in fruit and vegetable consumption in our diets.[7] Phytonutrients account for the vast array of colour in your fruit and vegetables. These colours are produced by the plant as a protective mechanism to stop predators from eating them while they are growing. These are particularly rich in plant food that has been grown organically as the plant will have had to mount its own defence rather than being sprayed with pesticides. Historically your hunter-gatherer ancestors would have eaten around eight hundred varieties. These 25,000 chemicals are powerful enough to switch DNA on and off when necessary to prevent and treat disease and transform your health.

By beginning **The In-Sync Diet** with a two-day cleanse rich in plant foods you will ensure that you are not falling short of vital nutrients to support your immune system, brain function and eye, bone and heart health as well as helping you to ditch the fat. You will continue a diet rich in whole foods, fruit and vegetables throughout the programme.

Top Tip: Aim to buy organic food if your budget allows Aim to ensure that as much of your food as possible is organic. This will help to minimise the number of toxic chemicals entering your body. The Soil Association is the UK's leading charity campaigning for healthy, humane and sustainable food, farming and land use. They provide information on their website on how to manage to buy organic food on a budget.

www.soilassociation.org/buyorganic/buyorganic/organic onabudget

Another reason for choosing organic food is that research indicates organic produce contains higher levels of certain nutrients compared with conventional produce. Basically, plant foods have to mount a defence to protect themselves against predators eating them before they are fully grown. It is the chemicals they produce to protect themselves that are of huge benefit to our health. Plant foods that have been sprayed with pesticides do not have to mount such a defence and, for this reason, are not as nutritious.

The Environmental Workers Group publishes a list of the fruit and vegetables most contaminated with pesticides and we have listed some below.[8] If you can, source the following organically:

1. Apples
2. Strawberries
3. Grapes
4. Celery
5. Peaches
6. Spinach
7. Sweet Bell Peppers
8. Nectarines
9. Cucumbers
10. Cherry Tomatoes
11. Sugar snap peas
12. Potatoes
13. Blueberries
14. Lettuce
15. Greens

Please note that fruit does not come into The In-Sync Diet until Phase Two.

Sauna therapy to support your two-day cleanse (OPTIONAL):

The skin is a major organ of elimination, but many of us do not sweat on a regular basis. Part of this problem may be due to our sedentary lifestyles and the wearing of synthetic or tight clothing.

Sauna - By allowing your skin to get hot for a matter of minutes, you can boil off a number of unwanted chemicals from fat under the skin. Visiting a sauna once per week may hugely benefit your health but do not think you need to last it out until you are practically passing out from heat exhaustion! Simply allowing your skin to glow may do.

Far Infrared Sauna - This is a great option because it heats your tissues that are several inches deep, enhancing your own metabolic processes and increasing your circulation. Unlike normal saunas, it heats you from the inside out rather than the other way around. This may mean that the elimination of toxins may be more effective. You can either book a session at a clinic that offers this service or hire/buy your own.

Sauna therapy is an effective method of cleansing and offers many health benefits.[8] Make sure that you rehydrate with plenty of water afterwards - see Chapter Three.

Please note that the success of your programme does **not** depend on you getting to a sauna - it is merely an optional extra to support good health. Working up a good sweat through exercise will also be extremely beneficial.

Footnotes

1. Madrigal A. http://www.wired.com/2009/09/humans-have-made-found-or-used-over-50-million-unique-chemicals/ 9th September 2009.
2. Neustadt J. and Piecenia S. A Revolution in Health: How to take charge of your health. 2008 J&S Media.

3. Department of Health and Human Services. Third National Report on Human Exposure to Environmental Chemicals. Atlanta, GA: Centers for Disease Control and Prevention; July 2005.

4. DiBaise J.K., Zhang H. et al. Gut microbiota and its possible relationship with obesity. *Mayo Clinic Proceedings.* Vol 83, issue 4, pp 460-469. April 2008.

5. Shishehbor F., Mansoori A. et al. Apple cider vinegar attenuates lipid profile in normal and diabetic rats. *Europe PubMed Central* 19630216 2008.

6. Wang X et al. Fruit and vegetable consumption and mortality from all causes, cardiovascular disease and cancer: a systemic review and dose-response meta-analysis of prospective cohort studies. *BMJ 2014*, 349: g4490.

7. Murphy M.M. et al. Global assessment of select phytonutrient intakes by level of fruit and vegetable consumption. *Br J Nutr* 11:1-15. 2014.

8. Crinnion W.J. Sauna as a valuable tool for cardiovascular, autoimmune, toxicant-induced and other chronic health problems. *Alternative Medicine Review: a journal of Clinical Therapeutic.* 16. (3):215-225 2011.

Chapter Six

Phase Two of The In-Sync Diet

Going Beyond Gluten and Lectins

Weeks One and Two

Congratulations you are now on Phase Two of the programme, which you will be following for the next two weeks. To make things easier for you, we have included a list of instructions that need to be followed on this part of the programme to ensure your success. Once you have got to grips with these instructions, you will then be taken through a list of what you can eat and what you need to avoid.

The Instructions for Phase Two:

Instruction number one:

Eat only three meals per day. It is actually no mean feat to cut food intake down to just three times per day because food is everywhere you go. We often do not register a lot of food we put into our mouths. We want you to eat breakfast, lunch and dinner for the duration of Phase Two and have nothing in between.

Glynis' Tip:

Before I met Fleur, I used to eat little and often. This meant that every afternoon I used to have a snack. The snack usually involved chocolate (dark and organic but still chocolate). I'm not going to lie, giving up snacking was hard. What's interesting, is that by not eating little and often but rather eating only at meal times with lots of protein and vegetables, makes you less hungry. Snacking is now a thing of the past for me. I rarely get hungry mid-afternoon and have no difficulty leaving 5 hours between meals. You too can do it, I promise.

Instruction number two:

Only have water or herbal teas/green tea/redbush tea (no milk or sugar) between meals. Anything that has calories will affect your ability to burn fat.

If you drink coffee and tea, you must have it with a meal rather than in between. If you smoke, you should try to have your cigarette after a meal not in between meals as this too can affect fat burn.

Instruction number three:

Have your fruit/nuts with meals. You can have two to three pieces of fruit but make sure you eat them at the end of meals or with a meal rather than in between.

Instruction number four:

Make sure you have some healthy protein with every meal. You will find a list of all the foods you can eat in the next section.

Instruction number five:

Include some vegetables with at least two and preferably three meals per day. Have a look at the previous chapter for the list of what you can eat.

Instruction number six:

Aim to finish your evening meal as early as possible - certainly no later than 9 pm.

Glynis' Tip:

For maximum benefit, eat dinner as early as possible. If I'm at home, I'll eat at about 6.30 or 7pm. If you go out, it's ok to eat a bit later occasionally. And yes it is possible to eat out at this stage of the diet. Just stick to protein and vegetables. Not difficult at all.

Instruction number seven:

Aim to leave five hours between meals. It is during these breaks between meals and whilst you sleep at night that a lot of the burning fat will take place.

Instruction number eight:

Please leave out alcohol for Phase Two - it may be put in at Phase Three.

Why we need to go beyond gluten

'The gut is not like Las Vegas. What happens in the gut does not stay in the gut.' Dr. Alessio Fasano, pioneering researcher on gluten and the gut and gastroenterologist.

Everyone is sensitive to wheat, or more specifically the protein gliadin found in gluten. Although we have been eating wheat for thousands of years, we are not engineered to digest gluten because we lack the 'machinery' or enzymes to do so. Gluten is what is known as an anti-nutrient because it interferes with your ability to absorb the nutrients from your food and can damage your intestinal tract. Gluten found in **wheat, barley** and **rye** tends to be the biggest culprit.

The reason it gives people so much trouble is that it is not broken down in the mouth and can arrive at the gut intact. Your gut covers the surface area of around 3,000 square feet which is about the size of a double tennis court. It is a huge gateway that protects your body from the outside world. Every day it has to deal with the onslaught of food, viruses, parasites and bacteria, as well as food additives, radiation, the list goes on.

What a fascinating new review article [1] has proven, beyond all doubt, is that gluten has the potential to leave gaping holes in your gut lining that can allow large food molecules into the bloodstream. These could cause unwanted reactions from your immune system. You also have a huge number of bacteria in your gut that normally work in your favour by helping you to digest your food and in producing vitamins and minerals, as well as antiviral and antibacterial substances. However, you want them to stay in the gut otherwise they can get into the bloodstream and hide anywhere. In their new locations they may not behave as well as they do in your intestine.

So many people tend to feel better on a gluten-free diet and can find that unexplained migraine headaches, body aches, dizziness and exhaustion just disappear.

Beyond gluten reducing your lectin load

The secret of success of **The In-Sync Diet** is that you will be going beyond gluten to reducing your lectin load. Lectins are proteins in foods that are anti-nutrients too and can also damage your gut.[2] Whilst it would be impossible to get them out of your diet completely, you can certainly make a difference by reducing them. **Gluten** (from wheat, barley and rye) belongs to this category as do **legumes** such as kidney beans and all the other beans that need soaking before cooking as well as lentils and chickpeas. They can cause you terrible discomfort such as indigestion, bloating, nausea and soreness known as inflammation.

A case in point

A while ago a hospital decided to have a 'healthy eating day' for the staff. Of course this is something they should focus on everyday but anyway, they picked a certain day and decided to serve chilli con carne. The chilli con carne was served but some of the staff noticed the kidney beans were still hard. Three hours later a registrar in the operating theatre started vomiting and soon many of the staff were doing the same. The problem was that the uncooked kidney beans had such a high lectin content that they made the staff ill.[3]

Lectins can make you fat

Lectins are trouble makers because they can also make you gain weight. They are able to do this because they are incredibly sticky and get stuck in places where they should not be. This has a knock-on effect of making you store more body fat. Lectins mimic your body's own hormones; the ones that are crucial for sending instructions to fat cells to tell them to either store more fat or to lay off for the time being. These disruptive proteins stick to the part of the cell where your hormones normally go and tell your cell to get fatter and fatter by taking in more and more energy! [4]

Glynis' Tip:

Even though gluten has often been blamed for causing gut problems, finding out that whole grains were not good (as explained in Chapter two) was a real shock. I knew that eating a lot of them would make you gain weight, but I presumed that eaten in moderation they were extremely healthful. And lentils??? The holy grail of vegetarians and health nuts everywhere! I was convinced I had misunderstood Fleur or that somehow she was mistaken. However, after having given up gluten and most grains and legumes a couple of years ago, I feel transformed. I thought it would be the hardest thing in the world, but it has been so much easier than I thought it would be. Having said that, I do occasionally indulge when I'm on my maintenance programme. I will sometimes eat (or even bake) gluten free cake as a special treat. Occasionally I'll have some rice or on the very odd occasion some bread, which I always try and keep gluten free. However, most of the time I have no grains at all and you know what? It's not that hard.

Foods you will be eating on The In-Sync Diet:

High Carbohydrate sources - no more than three to six tablespoons per day.

Please note: If you are smaller in build or you have not been particularly active in your day then three tablespoons will suffice. Only have six if you are of larger build or have been doing a couple of hours of exercise in your day. If you feel you can do without these starchy carbs but can eat loads of the vegetables below then do.

Beetroot	Pumpkin
Butternut squash	Swede
Carrots	Sweet potato
Parsnip	Turnip
Mandioca	Celeriac
Plantain	Tapioca

Protein sources - aim to have a piece of protein at least the size of the palm of your hand at each meal. A piece of fish the size of a cheque will be a meal portion.

White meat	Chicken, turkey, poussin, guinea fowl, duck, goose, quail, rabbit
Red meat (preferably grass-fed if you can)	Beef, lamb, pork
Fish and seafood	All varieties
Eggs	Chicken, duck, quail, goose 2 to 3 eggs would be a meal portion
Nuts	Almonds, walnuts, pecans, pinenuts, hazelnuts, pistachios can be added to meals to boost the protein content. Almond or cashew nut butter (A good handful would be a portion of nuts for the day or double that if you are using nuts as your only protein source at that meal.) (A tablespoon of nut butter would be a portion for the day or double that if you are using nuts as your only protein source at that meal.)
Traditionally fermented	Tofu or tempeh

Non-root vegetables (not including root vegetables above) are unlimited so try to get at least two to three 'mugs full' of a variety per day.

Artichokes	Greens: pak choy, Swiss chard, kale, spinach, mustard, beet greens
Asparagus	
Aubergine	Lettuce/mixed greens: romaine, red and green leaf, endive, spinach, rocket, radicchio, watercress, chicory
Bamboo shoots	
Bean sprouts	
Bell or other peppers	Mange tout
Broccoli	Mushrooms
Brussels sprouts	Okra
Cabbage (all types)	Radishes
Cauliflower	Salsa (sugar-free)
Celery	Sea vegetables (kelp, etc.)
Courgettes	Sugar snap peas
Chives, onion, leeks, garlic	Tomatoes/mixed vegetable juice
Cucumber	
Green Beans	Water chestnuts

To make the most of the healthy properties of vegetables aim to have the following each day:

- A portion from the cabbage family e.g. broccoli, cabbage, kale or cauliflower
- A variety of colour to get plenty of plant chemicals known as polyphenols.
- A portion from the onion family.
- Some salad leaves

Glynis' Tip:

As you will be eating no grains from now on, it's extremely important to eat an ample portion of vegetables each day. And the reason will quickly become apparent, trust me. Vegetables will supply the fibre you need to keep things moving…if you catch my drift…

The other thing is that you should never go hungry. There is no counting calories here or restricting portions (within reason). In fact, when I'm on the diet I sometimes struggle to eat the full amount of protein and vegetables Fleur demands. The important thing, however, is that you only eat the foods permitted and don't snack! You can take it from someone who was a major snacker, that you will adjust to this very quickly, as long as you are eating the right foods.

If you regularly eat grains and sugar, it will take your body a few days to get used to going without them. You may feel a little tired or even headachy to begin with but within a few days this will pass. The fact that you're allowed fat on this diet will help a lot and make it easier than other diets. If energy is low, do remember to have your portion of fruit with your meal. The first week is the hardest but very soon you will be feeling amazing and actually enjoying it. If you are struggling in the first few days, take it easy and remember it's only for a short time. Soon you will have energy levels you haven't had in years.

Fruit: 2 - 3 servings (see below)

Apple (1 medium)	Kiwi (2 medium)
Apricots (3 medium)	Mango (1/2 medium)
Berries: blackberries, blueberries, raspberries, strawberries (1 handful - approx 80g)	Nectarines (2 small)
Cantaloupe (1/2 medium)	Orange (1 large)
Cherries (15)	Peaches (2 small)
Fresh figs (2)	Pear (1 medium)
Grapefruit (1 whole)	Plums (2 small)
Grapes (15)	Tangerines (2 small)
Honeydew melon (74g small)	Watermelon (chopped, 2 handfuls)

Oils; extra virgin olive oil, olives, coconut oil, avocado oil and nut oils and avocado itself, organic (preferably grass fed) butter.

Coconut water/creamed coconut/coconut milk.

Seaweed e.g. Nori sheets and Arame (both Japanese seaweed products).

Beverages:

Coffee and tea can be drunk at mealtimes only.

Water (sparkling or still) in between meals or herbal teas/green tea/redbush tea without milk or sugar.

Herbs and spices:

Cinnamon, mustard, tamari sauce, apple cider vinegar, lime, lemon, flavoured extracts (vanilla or almond), fresh or dried herbs, pepper, fresh or dried chilli, ginger, garlic and spices.

Avoid sauces such as tomato ketchup and BBQ sauce

Foods to remove (high lectin load)
All grains (wheat, oats, barley, rye, millet, corn, rice, quinoa, buckwheat)
All dairy apart from organic butter (i.e. take out milk, cheese, yoghurt). Try almond milk or coconut milk instead.
All beans and legumes e.g. kidney beans, lentils, chickpeas, black beans, soya beans, PEANUTS are also in this category. Please note traditionally fermented soya such as tofu or tempeh is fine.
Potatoes
Peanuts
Seeds
Vegetable oils e.g. sunflower oil and corn oil
Dairy - milk, cheese, yoghurt
Sugar, dried fruit (apart from in the occasional food recipe) and fruit juices*
Convenience and processed foods (including margarine)*
Artificial sweeteners* e.g. in zero calorie drinks and squash and chewing gum
Alcohol - until Phase Three

Please note that if you eat legumes as part of your culture or you feel your diet would be too restricted without them, then very careful preparation is of the essence to remove as much of the lectin as possible.

Soak the beans for twelve hours in four times their weight in water and rinse thoroughly a few times. Then cook in fresh water until they are soft and rinse again. A pressure cooker can speed the cooking process up. A useful source of information on this can be found at www.westonprice.org/health-topics/putting-the-polish-on-those-humble-beans/

The trap of artificial sweeteners

When you eat sugar, a sensory area in your brain will be able to tell how many calories you have eaten and will induce a feeling of being full. Artificial sweeteners are many times sweeter than sugar and so the brain will expect to receive a certain number of calories, which it then doesn't get. The only answer, therefore, is to drive up appetite and cravings so the brain can get the energy it expected to have. Ironic but true, avoiding sugar by using artificial sweeteners or using 'low-calorie' or 'zero calorie' products will make you put on weight.[5]

What else to avoid between meals:

- Chewing gum - probably has been a part of our routine since time immemorial but nowadays it is made of synthetic rubber that has been infused with artificial sugars and flavourings.
- Flavouring for water such as juice or squash. Most squash contains either sugar or artificial sweeteners.
- Fizzy drinks.
- Coconut water - it may be a healthy drink, but it still contains sugar so keep for cooking only.

Dealing with withdrawal symptoms and food cravings

- Let go of the sugary foods and fizzy drinks and welcome a whole new world of tastes and textures.
- When you eat, try to sit down at a table rather than at your computer or on the sofa in front of the T.V. You begin eating your food with your brain which tells your gut to prepare for what is to come. You cannot do this if you are not mindfully eating.

- Enjoy the tastes, textures and flavours of the new foods you are eating. Chew each mouthful carefully.
- If you don't like a particular food - don't have it.
- Don't eat if you are stressed or anxious as you won't be able to digest your food. Your gastrointestinal tract has a direct link to the brain. Anxiety in the brain will also be felt in the gut and vice versa.
- Getting from one meal to another will be difficult at first but remember that your body *will* adjust and when it has, you have cracked it!
- When the cravings hit, concentrate all your thoughts on an alternative that gives you pleasure (preferably not something to do with food!).
- Make sure you are eating sufficient protein at meal times as this can keep you feeling fuller for longer.
- If you suffer from extreme blood sugar dips or are diabetic then please consult your medical practitioner before going on the programme.

Sample meal plan with three options:

Breakfast:

Berry breakfast	2 boiled eggs with steamed asparagus spears	1 piece of fish e.g. kipper or mackerel grilled and served with packet baby tomatoes

Five hours in between - water only

Lunch:

Please note: these suggestions are designed to give ideas for those of you who take your lunch to work or eat out. If you eat your lunch at home, then make it as nutritious as your evening meal.

Nori wraps (see recipe below) + packet baby tomatoes	Lettuce leaf wraps (see recipe below) + fruit	Omelette sandwich (see recipe below) + fruit

Five hours in between - water only

Dinner:

Creamed spinach and eggs + fruit	Green tea chicken soup + fruit	Fish creole + fruit

Sandwich wrap ideas to take to work

Lettuce leaf wraps - makes 4 wraps

8 large romaine lettuce leaves
8 slices cooked bacon
8 slices cooked chicken/turkey
4 slices tomatoes
1 sliced avocado
Chopped basil leaves
Gherkins – optional

Place 2 lettuce leaves on top of each other and sprinkle with chopped basil leaves.

Add 2 pieces of bacon, 2 slices turkey, slice of tomato and ¼ avocado.

Pull the lettuce leaves around the fillings and fasten together with a toothpick.

Cut in half.

Nori Wraps

Salmon steak mashed
1 carrot, peeled with a vegetable peeler into strands
Lettuce leaves (rocket, watercress, spinach)
1/2 avocado
Nori sheet
Tamari (gluten-free soy) sauce to taste

Pile it all in, roll it up and eat!
Swap ingredients as you wish.

Omelette Sandwiches

2 eggs, beaten
Pinch of salt
Pinch of ground pepper
1/2 teaspoon dried basil leaves
1 cup chopped ham
2 tablespoons butter

Combine eggs, salt, pepper, and basil in a large bowl and beat to blend; stir in ham. Heat the butter in non-stick pan and add egg mixture. Cook over medium heat 8-10 minutes, lifting edges of omelette occasionally to let uncooked portion flow under and cook until eggs are set. Remove from heat. Let sit for 2-3 minutes until cooled. Cut into quarters and put one-quarter on top of another to make a sandwich. Put slices of lettuce, tomato and cucumber in between.

Recipes

Berry Breakfast - serves 1

200g of frozen berries
150ml of coconut water (or until desired consistency)
1 tablespoon creamed coconut
1 tablespoon flaked roasted almonds
Handful of chopped kale (optional)
¼ of an avocado
Dash of vanilla extract

Blend all together in a food processor. Using frozen fruits eases the process and gives the smoothies a lovely texture and coolness. Fresh mango is also nice in smoothies. Most supermarkets do a variety of frozen fruits and berries.

Coconut Lime Plantain

1 plantain sliced
Pinch of salt
1 tablespoon of coconut oil
Half a lime

Lightly fry the plantain in coconut oil until golden brown. Add a little salt if desired and squeeze the lime over and serve. Alternatively, bake in the oven without oil and brush a little over for the last five minutes of cooking.

Green tea chicken casserole - serves 4-6

1 small free range organic chicken (1-1 ½ kg, any giblets removed)
4 large leeks
1 onion
8 medium carrots peeled
4 stalks celery
3 sprigs of thyme (or 1 teaspoon dried thyme)
2 bay leaves
1 large chunk of ginger (3-4cm) sliced
300ml strong green tea
A squeeze of lemon juice
3 tablespoons parsley chopped
Freshly ground pepper and a little sea salt

Wash the chicken and place in a large saucepan.

Cut the dark ends of the leeks and rinse under running water to remove any grit. Coarsely chop 2 leeks, setting the other 2 aside.

Coarsely chop 4 carrots, the onion, 2 celery stalks, 2-4 celery leaves and the ginger.

Put the chopped vegetables in the saucepan around the chicken along with ½ of the bay leaves and thyme. Fill saucepan with just enough water to cover the chicken. Bring to the boil, cover and simmer on the lowest heat for 1 ½ hours.

While the chicken is cooking, peel remaining carrots, quarter lengthwise and cube. Finely cube the remaining celery stalks and thinly slice the remaining leeks.

When the chicken is done, lift out of the stock and set aside to cool.

Sieve stock into another large saucepan and discard the first lot of vegetables.

Bring the stock to the boil again and add the remaining bay leaf, thyme and the finely chopped vegetables; first the carrots and celery, 5 minutes later the leeks.

Cook for another 5 minutes or until all vegetables are cooked, *al dente*.

While the vegetables are cooking, remove the chicken skin and discard. Shred the meat and set aside.

When vegetables are cooked, add green tea and meat, and reheat gently for 2-3 minutes. Season with pepper, salt, lemon, lemon zest and ginger. Scatter with parsley and serve with lots of extra vegetables.

Mexican Style Scrambled Tofu - serves 1

200g tofu
1 cup of chopped tomato, courgette, onion
1 tablespoon of olive oil
1 teaspoon mixed herbs
Tabasco sauce
Cracked pepper and sea salt to taste
Paprika

Put the oil in the pan on low heat and add chopped vegetables. Sauté with herbs for five minutes until soft. Add the tofu and break up in the pan. Season with paprika and salt and pepper to taste. Serve with Tabasco on the side.

Fish Creole - serves 4

1 tablespoon extra virgin olive oil
1 onion chopped
110g thin-sliced celery
55g green pepper chopped
1 garlic clove finely chopped
2 tablespoons fresh parsley (or 2 teaspoon dried)
1 bay leaf
¼ teaspoon rosemary chopped
1 800g tinned tomatoes
450g fish fillets

Heat oil in a large saucepan and lightly sauté the onion, celery, pepper and garlic until soft.

Add parsley, bay leaf, rosemary and tomatoes.

Simmer uncovered for about 20 minutes.

Add fish fillets in small pieces and simmer until cooked through, about 5 - 10 minutes.

Remove bay leaf. Serve with cauliflower rice.

Healthy Cauliflower Rice Recipe - this is a great alternative to rice

1 cauliflower cut into florets
2 teaspoons of extra-virgin olive oil
½ cup diced white onion
1 clove garlic crushed
½ cup of water

Grate the cauliflower florets into grain-like pieces. This can be done either with a food processor with a grating attachment or a cheese grater.

Heat the oil in a wok or frying pan. Add the garlic and onion and sauté for five minutes.

Add the water and cover for five minutes. The cauliflower should be cooked and the water absorbed.

Creamed spinach & eggs - serves 1

1 large handful of fresh spinach chopped (well-drained frozen spinach can also be used)
2 tablespoons of lightly roasted cashew nuts ground to a fine powder
1 tablespoon coconut oil
A little water
A pinch of nutmeg
Sea salt
3 poached eggs

Melt the coconut oil in a pan and add the spinach, cook until the spinach is softened. Meanwhile, add a little water to the cashew nut powder to form a creamy paste. Add the paste to the spinach and warm through on a low heat. Add the sea salt and nutmeg. Serve with the three poached eggs on top.

Glynis' Tip:

There are lots of simple options for meals as well.

Lunch:

A staple of mine is smoked salmon. I eat the entire packet with a salad of mixed vegetables including avocado and olives. Followed by fruit (A favourite is mango. Fresh coconut chunks are great too when a sugar craving hits. I usually have some with my fruit but not in between meals.).

Salad Nicoise - a tin of tuna with salad and 2 boiled eggs. Very filling and satisfying.

Dinner:

Fish (cod or any white fish) - rub with olive oil and slice on some favourite vegetables. I like leeks, capers and olives piled on top. Place in oven at 200 degrees for 30 minutes.

Or pour on tamari sauce with chopped ginger. This works well with salmon.

A lovely satisfying side is sweet potato fries. I soften a spoonful of coconut oil in the oven, cut the sweet potato into chips, mix with the oil and season with a bit of pink Himalayan or sea salt. Bake in the oven for 30 minutes at 200 degrees. However, keep your portion quite small (about ½ of a sweet potato).

And then there are stir fries. Chop up whatever vegetables you have to hand (I always include either an onion or leek) and add prawns or chicken cubes. Also chopped ginger (I always have fresh ginger in my fridge) and maybe some cashew nuts. Add tamari sauce at end.

***NB** I use tamari as opposed to soy sauce because it's wheat free.*

Footnotes

1. Fasano A. Intestinal permeability and its regulation by zonulin: diagnostic and therapeutic implications. *Clin Gastroenterol Hepatol*, 10(10): 1096-1100. 2012.
2. Freed DLJ. Lectins in food: their importance in health and disease. *J Nutr Med*, 2:45-64. 1991.

3. Freed DLJ. Do dietary lectins cause disease? BMJ 318:1023-4, 1999.
4. Jonsson et al. Agrarian diet and diseases of affluence. Do evolutionary and novel lectins cause leptin resistance. *BMS Endocr Disord*. 5:10 2005.
5. Feijo F. de M. et al. Saccharin and aspartame, compared with sucrose, induce greater weight gain in adult Wistar rats at similar total caloric intake levels. *Appetite* 60(1) 203-7. January 2013.

Chapter Seven

Getting Moving on an Empty Stomach

A lot of us set the intention to follow a regular exercise routine, start off and then give up after a week or two. On The In-Sync Diet, the key is to slowly build activity into your daily life rather than viewing it as an obligation that needs to be undergone a couple of times per week. **The beauty of it is that you do not need to get to the gym to be active.**

- We recommend that you start off by incorporating thirty to forty minutes of brisk movement into your day to get your heart rate up.
- After that you can start adding in some High-Intensity Exercise (see below), which takes up very little time but is very effective in helping you regain your muscle tone and burn fat.

Getting your heart rate up

Getting your heart rate up will improve your physical fitness and help you to lose weight. Your heart rate is calculated by the number of times your heart beats in a minute (BPM). The best time to measure your resting heart rate is in the morning before you get out of bed when you are more relaxed - unless you have overslept!

- Put your fingers on either your wrist or your neck to feel your pulse and make a note of the number of times you feel a beat to get your resting heart rate. Typically it will be between sixty to a hundred BPM but this can be lower in fitter people.
- Now try and go about a daily activity such as the vacuuming, mowing, clearing out the garden shed or walking to the train station at a brisker pace than normal until you feel yourself slightly out of breath. This is a very simple way of improving your fitness. You can then put your fingers to your pulse to see how different activities will increase your heart rate.
- It is important that your heart rate comes back down after exercise so sit and enjoy some delicious food and think calming thoughts.

- When you try the High-Intensity exercises later on in this chapter, you can work towards doing them at a pace where you cannot speak more than a few words.

Top Tip:

You might also like to measure your movement with a pedometer to become more mindful of the amount of activity you do in a day. **Pedometers** count electronic pulses each time you take a step. Sedentary people will typically take around three thousand steps per day whilst active people can reach ten thousand.[1] Aim to reach at least five thousand and then gradually increase this by following these recommendations:

- Take the stairs instead of the lift.
- Always walk the long way round to where you are going.
- Meet up with a friend for a walk instead of coffee.
- Walk between offices rather than using the phone.
- Extend your daily walks with the dog.

How to become a 'fat-burner' not a 'sugar-burner'

Did you know that your genes have barely changed since the Stone Age? What this means for you is that you can be super fit and lean just like your Palaeolithic ancestors! The In-Sync Diet will show you their secrets.

On The In-Sync Diet we would like you to build activity into your daily life in a way that your ancestors would have done. We want you to start to move around *before you have eaten*! This may feel completely strange at first and not at all what you are used to doing. We talked in Chapter One about how it is your brain that regulates your metabolism because it is the most energy-greedy organ of all. When you are feeling the first signs of hunger, this is your signal to move and your brain will take care of the rest.[2] So go on, see how it feels.

Moving around on empty

Your Stone Age ancestors did not eat before they set off in the morning and you do not need to either! When you move before you eat, your body has all sorts of clever ways of getting the energy it needs and one of these is by burning fat! We will only burn fat if there really is no other alternative. The problem is that in our modern society food is all around. By constantly putting food into our mouths, whether it is high-calorie or low-calorie, our body will only burn sugar. To become a 'fat-burner', you need to 'forage' first then eat.

What this means in practical terms is that instead of grabbing the cereal before you do the school run or go to work, just go out. Go to your exercise class or walk around the park then eat afterwards when you have the opportunity to 'rest and digest'.

Not eating before exercise is the key to burning fat. The more you are able to do this, the better control you will have of your blood sugar levels and the less prone you will be to putting on weight. So remember move first then eat, rest and digest.

Be confident that even if this is difficult at first, your metabolism will reset itself and within a couple of weeks your body will be used to it. You can do it!

Glynis' Tip:

Ok, exercise is where I come into my own. I swear by it. I talk about it at every given opportunity and write about it on my anti-ageing website all the time.

As I always say "Exercise is the closest thing there is to an Anti-Ageing Pill".

If you want to lose weight and look your very best at whatever age you are, then exercise is the key.

As Fleur explains, there are many reasons for this. If you already exercise, you will know the feel good buzz you get from it. If you never exercise or are one of those who have an aversion to it, then clearly this is going to be more of a challenge.

Start easy, in this case. Just adding a brisk walk is going to make a difference. Try going to a Pilates class or a Zumba class.

For me, exercise has been a life saver. It's the time of the day that's just for me. All troubles are forgotten, all chores are put aside. Stress dissolves away. Muscles become toned and lean.

Think of it as a gift to yourself rather than a punishment. You will be amazed at how different you will look and feel.

Having said that, when Fleur first suggested I exercise on an empty stomach having skipped breakfast, I was horrified. Firstly, I love breakfast and secondly, I was convinced I would faint...or possibly die. The thought of going to the gym or my hot yoga class with no food inside me actually scared me. Fleur seemed unfazed by my fear and declared I would adjust very quickly. I told her to have the paramedics on standby.

So after a lifetime of enthusiastic breakfast eating, I began to skip it and….gulp….do exercise. The first hot yoga session, I did feel a little light headed, but that was it. To my complete and utter amazement, within a week it was as if I had never had breakfast in my life. I exercised normally and lived to tell the tale. I stopped wanting breakfast and now rarely feel hungry when I wake up. However, on the odd occasion I do wake up hungry or if I'm not going to exercise that morning, I do eat breakfast. It all works rather well. And I'm a lot fitter than I was before. (At this stage you are still eating breakfast, albeit, after your exercise. This will help prepare you for missing it altogether on occasions at a later phase.)

Suggestions for how to add in some basic High-Intensity exercises into your daily routine alongside daily movement:

If you already have an exercise regime, then you should carry on. If you are new to exercise, once you have trained yourself to go about your everyday activities at a brisker pace then you can move on to the following exercises.

LEVEL ONE: Beginner

Do some basic exercise just before eating - five to ten minutes only.

Just before **at least one** of the three meals of the day, you should do the following:

Either:

A.   Walk/run up and down stairs ten times
Or:

B.   Do twenty sit-ups, forty push-ups and forty squats.
Or:

C.   Ten Burpees

How to perform a Burpee

1.   Start in a standing position and drop into a squat position (as if you're sitting back in a chair) with your hands on the ground.
2.   Bring your palms to the floor and extend your feet back in one quick motion to assume the front plank position.
3.   Return to the squat position in one quick motion.
4.   Return to an upright standing position.

How to Modify the Burpee

If it's too challenging at first, here's a simple modification: Instead of going into plank position, do a Burpee by a wall. Squat down, stand up and do a push-up against a wall. (This is especially important for anyone with knee or shoulder issues.)

High-Intensity Interval Training (HIIT) on an empty stomach

High-Intensity Interval Training is a fantastic way of exercising when you are short of time. And not only that, it will really help you burn fat. The way it works is that your session should be short in duration but intense i.e. difficult enough to raise the heart rate to get you to the point that you cannot really say very much. A twelve-week study using HIIT on overweight young males showed that by doing a twenty-minute session three times per week, they were able to significantly reduce their body fat. Not only that they're visceral fat which is the dangerous fat around the organs, reduced by 17% and their aerobic capacity significantly increased.[3]

And there is even more good news! By doing a high-intensity interval training on an empty stomach, you will be encouraging your brain to work at optimum capacity. This means that you will be burning fat and getting smarter at the same time! [4]

You may find the morning the perfect time to do the following exercises.

Leave half an hour after you finish before you eat to maximise your fat burning potential.

Typical 20-minute interval session - running or cycling

1. 3 minute warm-up.
2. Interval 1: 30 seconds high intensity followed by 30 seconds at medium intensity (total time 1 minute).
3. Recover: 2 minutes.
4. Repeat interval and recovery sequence at least a further 7 times.
5. 3 minute cool down.

Stretch all used muscle groups thoroughly after (but not before) exercising. Typically this might take 5 or more minutes.

Please note that this can be done whether you are at home, outside or even in the office. A few minutes of exercise before eating (before at least two meals of the day) is an essential part of the programme. We challenge you to do it at work!

LEVEL TWO: Intermediate seven-minute exercise

Once you are beginning to find the exercises in Level One too easy, then you can progress on to Level Two. The beauty of doing the following exercises is that you will be working both your aerobic and anaerobic systems to really improve body tone and fitness. Level Two encourages you to reap the benefits of what is known as *High-Intensity Circuit Training*. High-Intensity Circuit Training incorporates fitness and resistance work to really increase your fat burning potential.

HICT SAMPLE PROGRAM from the American College of Sport's Medicine's Health and Fitness Journal [5]

All exercises can be done wherever you are (*e.g.*, home, office, hotel room, etc.) using nothing but your own body weight, a chair and a wall. The programme is a total body workout.

Because it needs to be performed at a high intensity, you should perform each exercise for 30 seconds and then rest for only ten seconds before going to the next station. Total time for the entire circuit workout should be approximately 7 minutes. The circuit can be repeated 2 to 3 times.

Please be warned that this is an intensive exercise and you may want to become familiar with each of the exercises first before attempting the whole circuit.

1. **Jumping jacks** (Total body) - jump raising your arms in the air and separating your legs to the side. Then jump again bringing your arms back down by your side and your legs back together.

2. **Wall sit** (Lower Body) - stand up against a wall with your feet at shoulder width apart, about 2 feet away from the wall. Gradually slide your back down the wall until your thighs are parallel to the ground, holding your arms out in front of you. (Make sure your knees are above your ankles and not over your toes.)

3. **Push-up** (Upper body) - kneel on the floor and put your arms out in front of you with your hands flat on the floor at shoulder-width apart. Stretch your legs out behind you and squeeze your bottom and tighten your stomach to make a line with your body. Slowly lower yourself down until your elbows are bending at a 90 degree angle, keeping them close to your body. Then push back up to your original position.

4. **Abdominal crunch** (Core) - lie down on your back with your knees bent up and your feet flat on the floor. Bring your hands behind your neck and interlink your fingers at the back of your neck. Take a deep breath and as you exhale use the strength of your abdomen to lift your head and shoulders up. Exhale and lower your head and shoulders to the floor.

5. **Step-up onto chair** (Total body) - place a chair in front of you and stand with your feet at hip-width apart with your arms by your side. Step onto the seat of the chair with one foot and then bring the other foot up next to it. Then step down with the foot you started with and bring the other foot back down next to it. Then next time begin with the opposite foot making sure you are keeping your stomach muscles tight and your back straight.

6. **Squat** (Lower body) - stand up with your feet slightly wider than shoulder-width apart. Hold your arms so that they are bent at the elbow and your palms are facing inwards. Breathe in and push your bottom out as you bend your knees. Keep your back straight and your chest and shoulders up as you go down making sure your knees are in line with your

feet. Breathe out and push your heels down as you go back up keeping the balls of your feet on the ground.

7. **Triceps dip on chair** (Upper body) - sit on the edge of the seat of the chair with your feet together, resting on your heels. Put your hands on the edge of the seat on either side of your thighs. Bend your elbows at 90 degrees and lower yourself down towards the floor. Then raise your body back up to the start by straightening your arms.

8. **Plank** (Core) - Start in the push-up position (as in picture 3). Lower your forearms down so your elbows and fists are touching the ground. Hold your fists together underneath the line of your shoulders. Imagine you are a plank of wood by engaging your stomach muscles and keeping your body straight. Hold this position keeping your glance to the floor in front of you.

9. **High knees/running in one place** (Total body) - run in one place raising one leg at a time lifting it up as high off the floor as you can. At the same time raise

the opposite arm i.e. if your right leg is lifted you should raise your left arm and vice versa.

10. **Lunge** (Lower body) - stand up straight with your legs hip-width apart and engage your stomach muscles. Then take a step forward with your right foot keeping your arms by your side. Keep your back straight as your body moves forward and bend both knees at the same time. Make sure your right knee does not go over your toe line. Then push off your right heel to come back up again to the starting position. Repeat with the left leg.

11. **Push-up and rotation** (Upper body) - start in a push-up position (as in picture 3) and then shift your body weight onto one side. Rotate your body and raise your arm. Return back to push-up position and repeat on the other side.

12. **Side plank** (Core) - lie on your right side with your legs stretched out. Then prop your upper body up using your right elbow and forearm. Raise your hips until your body forms a straight line and hold.

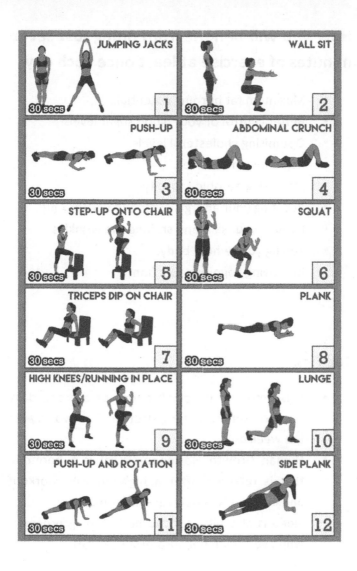

How you will benefit from doing just seven minutes of exercise at least once each day

- Maximum fat burning potential.
- Better control of your blood sugar levels.
- Optimising cholesterol levels.
- Regulating hormones.
- Increasing aerobic capacity.
- Boosting your energy levels and your sex life.
- Firming your skin and shifting the wrinkles.
- Toning your whole body.
- Improving cognitive function.

Top Tips:

- It is better to do small bursts of exercise daily than to exercise in long stretches on two days of the week only.
- Human Growth Hormone (HGH) is a hormone that is released after a high-intensity workout and is linked to a decrease in fat mass.
- Sleep is also vital for the body toning process - when you sleep you also produce HGH.

Footnotes

1. Bohannan R.W. Number of pedometer-assessed steps taken per day by adults: a descriptive meta-analysis. *Phys Ther* 2007 Dec; 87(12) 1642-50.
2. Peters A, Pellerin L et al. Causes of obesity: Looking beyond the hypothalamus. *Progress in Neurobiology,* Volume 81, Issue 2, Feb 2007, Pages 61-88.
3. Heydari M. et al. The effect of high-intensity intermittent exercise on the body composition of overweight males. *Journal of Obesity* January 2012.
4. Ferris L.T. et al. The effect of acute exercise on serum brain-derived neurotrophic factor levels and cognitive function. *Medicine and Science in Sports and Exercise* 39(41)) 728-734 2007.
5. Klika B. High-Intensity Circuit Training Using Body Weight. *ACSM's Health and Fitness Journal.* Vol 17, Issue 3, pp 8-13, May/June 2013.

Chapter Eight

Phase Three - Weeks three and four

Congratulations you are about to start the third phase of The In-Sync Diet programme. You are even further along your way to becoming a 'fat burner' rather than a 'sugar-burner'! At this stage, you may want to hop back on the scales to see how you are doing or you may be able to tell the difference simply by feeling how your clothes are fitting you.

Remember that you should be weighing your body fat and not your body weight. Your total body water should also have increased.

You will be resetting your metabolism by eating less frequently and exercising on an empty stomach. Not only are you bringing energy and vitality back into your life by burning fat, you are also working towards being in a state of optimal health. So let's have a look at the programme so far...

Summary of The In-Sync Diet so far:

- Drink enough water i.e. drink plenty to quench your thirst when you feel that you might be thirsty and don't drink again until you are - see Chapter Three.

- Don't snack or put anything into your mouth between meals apart from water! What this means is, don't have anything in between meals that will stop you burning fat. You should only be having water/green tea/red bush tea without sugar or milk between meals. The same goes for after dinner - once you have finished your evening meal, don't go back into the kitchen!

- Aim to leave five hours between your three meals as this is the magic time where you will be burning fat. Any disturbance will prevent this from happening.

- Always eat protein with your vegetables/fruit at each meal.

- Minimise starchy carbs I.e. root vegetables. (Potatoes, pasta, bread, etc...are not included in The In-Sync Diet.)

- Use healthy fats every day like cold pressed unfiltered virgin olive oil, coconut oil (to keep you fuelled for longer), omega-3 fats from oily fish and undamaged saturated fats from grass-fed meats.

- 'Eat a rainbow every day' to boost your phytonutrient intake - go for as much colour variety in your fruit and vegetable choices as you can.
- Add in some short bursts of movement/high-intensity movement before you eat your first meal of the day as hunger should be the signal to move not to eat. This could simply be walking to work or taking the kids to school, but it should be at a pace that you feel your heart rate (slightly) raised.
- Eat one to three servings of fruit per day with meals, not in between.

Instructions for Phase Three

'Most diets have focused on what to eat rather than looking at when not to eat.'
Dr. Robert Verkerk, scientific director of The Alliance for Natural Health International and www.bitethesun.org.

Instruction One:

Putting the 'pulling power' back into your day by skipping breakfast

Eat only three meals per day but **on two to three days per week, eat only two**. This is probably easiest done by skipping breakfast and having a late brunch. By doing this, you are engaging in a practice known as 'intermittent fasting' which literally means occasionally not eating. Intermittent fasting has been shown to be a much more effective weight loss strategy than calorie control.

You have already been introduced to this practice in the previous chapter. Moving around before you eat is really a form of intermittent fasting. And moving around before you eat will encourage your body to make some energy by burning fat. In this chapter, The In-Sync Diet is taking you a stage further by encouraging you to leave twelve to eighteen hours before your next meal after an overnight fast.

Glynis' Tip:

As I mentioned previously in Chapter 7, giving up breakfast came as a shock. However, I think it's much more of a mental adjustment than a physical one (it literally took me less than a week to adjust to having no breakfast at all). Most of us are firmly entrenched in our view of breakfast being the most important meal of the day. I would say this is the most fundamental difference I have made to the way I eat and the benefits have been huge. And trust me, I LOVED my breakfast! However, it's not a case of never ever having breakfast again. I love having pancakes sometimes or a big hearty breakfast... and I do...but only occasionally. Most days I start by exercising and then have lunch. If I'm very hungry, lunch will be early, but my body is now so adjusted to this way of eating that often when I'm busy, lunch is quite late. The good thing is you only have to do this 2 or 3 times a week for the moment, so not too hard. I went cold turkey and gave up breakfast completely when I first met Fleur. Whenever you are tempted to scoff your cereal or toast, just think of all the fat that will be burning off if you skip it!

Top Tip to get past the hunger pangs:

If you have a sedentary job, aim to get up from the chair every forty-five minutes perhaps to drink some water. If you are feeling motivated, you could even run up and down stairs a few times! You will be getting rid of those hunger pangs and cravings by doing so.

Instruction Two:

On the days you are only eating two meals per day aim to have half a plate of good quality protein (refer to Chapter Six) and the other half of vegetables. The vegetables may be steamed, sautéed, roasted or eaten raw with a dressing made from olive oil and apple cider vinegar.

Instruction Three:

Eat your high starch vegetables with the evening meal and this will mean that they are less likely to be stored as fat around the waist. Your evening meal, therefore, may be slightly bigger. This may be in complete contrast to what you have always been led to believe. But new research is showing that eating slightly later on, rather than in the early part of the day, is better for burning fat.[2]

Instruction Four:

On the days when you are not eating two meals per day follow the points in the summary overleaf.

Instruction Five:

Moderate alcohol consumption may be reintroduced if you wish. Please note that it is better to have it with meals as any alcohol that is drunk in the gaps between meals may interrupt the fat-burning potential. It should only be wine or spirits to reduce your lectin load (See Chapter Six).

Glynis' Tip:

For me personally, introducing alcohol into the equation seriously undermines my dieting efforts. Being on a maintenance programme is another thing, but if you are keen to really lose weight and get into great shape, I would highly recommend staying off the booze for as long as possible. Alcohol tends to give you a devil may care attitude and it becomes so much easier to cheat. I always want to eat more when I drink. However, you may be more disciplined than me and being allowed to drink may even encourage you to stay on the diet. In which case, go ahead but do try and stick to one glass at this stage of the diet.

Case Study:

Susan forgot to set her alarm for the next day and was woken up by the dog barking downstairs. Her husband was angry because he would be late for his meeting. Susan rushed out of bed to get the kids ready for school - they were grumpy at being rushed. Susan then had to get herself to work wondering what she was going to say to her boss. On her way to the station, she grabbed herself a couple of pastries and coffee because she was worried she was going to faint with hunger.

At this point, the brain has no 'pulling power' because Susan is out-of-sync. To compensate for this, she eats every few hours to keep her blood sugar levels going. By the time she gets home in the evening she is exhausted and hungry even though she has managed to consume a tremendous amount of high-calorie foods all day.

Why breakfast may not be the best meal of the day

There is a shared belief that breakfast is the meal that is most necessary because it sets you up for the day. But what it has the capacity of doing is setting you up for a roller coaster ride of unstable blood sugar levels. This is all to do with a hormone called cortisol, which is an activity hormone. It promotes activity as part of a necessary 'stress' reaction to get you going in the morning. It ensures that you have the energy to be ready for action by allowing the release of sugar into the bloodstream. Cortisol is an 'activity' hormone meaning that hunger should be what makes us move rather than a signal to sit down and eat. By eating at 'breakfast' time, you may be flooding your system with too much energy that has to be packed away very quickly. It is this that will create the hunger pangs later on. By skipping breakfast you are relying on your brain's 'pulling power' and this is a much more effective means of increasing your energy levels because you will be burning fat.

Glynis' Tip:

If your work schedule does not allow you to do any form of exercise in the morning, it may be best to have breakfast and then fast during the day by skipping lunch.

It would be ideal to then do a workout before your evening meal. The best way to get through the day like this is to have a slightly later breakfast. Remember that by exercising on an empty tummy, you will be burning fat.

Top Tip:

New research shows that your genes are not suited to frequent eating. Eating too frequently can upset the way your genes are expressed. This can have a devastating effect on your weight and your health.[2] By eating two or three times only per day and making healthy food choices from The In-Sync Diet, you will be toned and lean and feeling fantastic too.

Breakfast is also a time of day when you tend to eat food with a heavy lectin-load (see Chapter Six) that can really interfere with your weight loss intentions. The market is flooded with breakfast cereals - wheat-based, gluten-free, wholegrain, with chocolate, with cinnamon, with dried fruit - none of which are going to help you lose weight. Not having breakfast has been associated with the following benefits:

- You will feel less hungry throughout the day.
- You will be eating less throughout the day.

- You will be burning more fat.
- You will not suffer so many food cravings.
- Your brain will function better (see Getting Moving - Phase Three).
- Your blood sugar levels will be more stable.

Sample meal plan for two meals per day:

Brunch/Lunch:

Day one	Day two	Day three
Salmon steak(s) with Swiss chard sautee (see below) and fruit	Morning oven tomatoes (see below) and a three egg omlette with mushrooms, smoked salmon and fruit	Chicken broth with braised chicken breast and vegetable spirals (see below) and fruit

You may be leaving up to seven hours or more in between - water only

Dinner:

Day one	Day two	Day three
Sweet potato frittata (see below) with salad and fruit	Sword fish caponata + steamed vegetables and fresh tomato sauce Fruit	Chicken tagine Shaved fennel and Granny Smith salad

Glynis - These recipes are by my dear friend Gina To, who is a wonderful and inspirational cook. Enjoy!

Recipes

Sweet Potato Frittata with Toasted Almonds - Serves three to four

As I was trying out my new mandoline, this dish came together in just minutes. You can hand slice with just a little more time, but I promise the result is surprisingly sweet, salty and savoury.

1/3 cup olive oil
1 small yellow onion sliced thin
1 large sweet potato sliced thin
1 handful toasted almond slices
10 eggs beaten
Sea salt/cracked pepper

Preheat oven to 180c/350f.

Large non-stick ovenproof frying pan.

Heat olive oil.

Sauté onion and potatoes on medium heat until the potatoes are fork tender. Add half the almonds. Do not brown. Generously salt and pepper potato mixture.

In a medium sized bowl.

Beat eggs and add a bit more salt and pepper.

Pour tender potato and onion mixture into a bowl with the eggs and then pour it all back into the pan.

Cook on low for 10 minutes or until bottom sets

Remove from heat and place in a hot oven until top of eggs set (another 3 minutes).

Watch carefully so not to overcook.

Sprinkle with a few more almonds and serve, hot, warm, or cold. Delicious!!

Fresh Tomato Sauce

1/3 cup olive oil
5 cloves garlic chopped
1 bunch fresh basil (1/2-3/4 cup) chopped
2 cups chopped tomatoes fresh
1/4 teaspoon salt
1/4 teaspoon pepper
1 teaspoon red pepper flakes (optional)

In a medium size pot heat oil, sauté garlic and red pepper. Add the tomatoes, basil, salt and pepper. Cook uncovered for 20-25 minutes.

Swiss Chard Sauté

An earthy delight straight from the heavens. Cook it low and slow for a long time.

Avocado oil or olive oil
2 Shallots sliced
1 bunch Swiss Chard chopped
2 twigs thyme
2 bell peppers sliced
5 Cremini mushrooms sliced
Handful of toasted almonds

Heat 3 tablespoons plus a little more oil in the pan.

Throw in shallots and sauté for about 3 minutes. Add bell peppers, thyme, salt and pepper. Cook for 15 minutes. Add mushrooms and cook low and slow until all veggies are soft and melded together about 20-30 minutes. Add Swiss chard and sauté until wilted.

Salt and pepper to taste.

Sprinkle with toasted almonds and serve.

Goes great alongside chicken or fish. Feel free to drizzle a little olive oil or balsamic vinegar before serving.

Celeriac Crunch Salad

When I go to Paris, an overwhelming force hustles me into La Bon Marche Food Hall directly to the celeriac salad! Their fresh crunchy creamy goodness is like a magnet! The tenderness of the celeriac makes this "French Coleslaw" unforgettable.

Here is my best shot!

1 lemon juiced
Zest of 1 small orange
1 head celeriac grated
1 head fennel grated
2 teaspoons Dijon mustard
3 teaspoons mayo
3 tablespoons olive oil (more if needed)
Salt
Cracked pepper
1 tablespoon fresh chopped parsley

In a small bowl combine mustard, mayo, olive oil and lemon and zest - whisk until incorporated.

Add salt and pepper to taste (don't be shy).

Pour over grated veggies.

Toss well and refrigerate for at least 2 hours before serving.

Sprinkle with parsley before serving.

Morning Oven Tomatoes

1 packet of cherry tomatoes
3 tablespoons olive oil
Sprinkle of garlic powder
1 teaspoon basil chopped
1 teaspoon fresh parsley chopped
Salt
Pepper
Toasted almonds

I love baking tomatoes.

Preheat oven 180/350f.

Place the tomatoes in a baking dish. Pour olive oil over the top. Add the garlic powder, parsley and basil and season well with salt and pepper. Mix thoroughly with hands coating tomatoes well with all ingredients.

Sprinkle with almonds over the top.

Drizzle top lightly with olive oil.

Bake for 20-25 minutes.

Serve hot.

This dish goes well with eggs.

Chicken Tagine - Serves four

This recipe is simple yet it delivers the complicated flavours of a pro.

3 tablespoons of olive oil
1 whole chicken cut up
2 large shallots sliced (yellow onion good too)
3 figs halved
2 bell peppers sliced
2 cups chicken broth
2 zucchini or courgettes cut into 1" rounds
2 carrots cut into ½" rounds
2 teaspoons fresh parsley chopped
2 Tablespoons fresh cilantro or coriander chopped
1 teaspoon sea salt
1 teaspoon black pepper
1 teaspoon ginger powder
1 teaspoon turmeric
1 teaspoon cinnamon
5 dried apricots quartered

In a large pan, coat chicken in olive oil. Top with shallots. Sprinkle with salt, pepper, ginger powder, turmeric and cinnamon.

Cover and cook on medium-high for 15 minutes.

Add broth, carrots, zucchini, bell peppers, parsley, figs, apricots and cilantro. Cover and cook until chicken falls off the bone, about 30 more minutes.

Serve it over cauliflower rice - see Chapter Six.

Chicken Bone Broth

12 cups filtered water
1 chicken carcass and giblets
1 tablespoon apple cider vinegar
1 onion chopped
3 large carrots chopped
4 cloves crushed garlic
2 celery stalks
2 bay leaves
1 teaspoon Himalayan salt
½ teaspoon of freshly ground black pepper
1 bunch fresh parsley

Put the water and chicken parts in a slow cooker or saucepan with a lid and cook on high heat for two hours. Skim off the foam on the surface and turn down the heat. Add the remaining ingredients apart from the parsley and cook on low for about twelve hours. (Please note if you do not have a slow cooker you may need to do this over the course of two days.) Turn off the pot, take off the top layer of fat and stir in the parsley. Leave with the lid on for a further thirty minutes. Strain through a sieve and eat or store in the fridge/freezer for later use. This lengthy cooking time helps to remove as many minerals and nutrients as possible from the bones. By the end, so many minerals will have leached from the bones into the broth that the bones should crumble when pressed lightly between your thumb and forefinger.

Top Tip: Bone broths are anti-ageing

Bone broths are incredibly rich in nutrients. They also support the body's detoxification process and are used to make haemoglobin, bile salts and other naturally occurring chemicals within the body. They are rich in gelatine which improves the collagen status, thus supporting skin health. Gelatine also supports digestive health. And last but not least, bone broths are Nature's best antibiotic; they help mitigate the side effects of colds, flus and upper respiratory infections.

How to braise a chicken breast

Braising is a method of cooking where you brown the main ingredient (it does not have to be chicken, it can be meat, fish or vegetables) in oil and then add some bone broth so that the meat (or another ingredient) is just about covered in the pan. Add a lid and allow to simmer until cooked through. You will find the results are deliciously tender.

Top Tip: Buy yourself an inexpensive spiral vegetable slicer to create your own raw food vegetable noodles. Make courgette and carrot spirals and add to your bone broth and braised chicken at the serving stage.

Alternatively serve with a large mixed salad on the side.

Shaved Fennel and Granny Smith Salad

8 baby tomatoes
1 bulb fennel shaved
½ Granny Smith apple peeled and julienned
2-3 tablespoons olive oil
¼ orange plus zest
Sea salt
Fresh cracked black pepper

In a small pot with 2 cups of water. Add tomatoes and cook for 2 minutes.

Prepare a small bowl of water with ice cubes.

Remove tomatoes from boiling water and blanch them in the ice water.

Remove the skins from tomatoes, cut each one in half, and set aside.

In a salad bowl add the fennel, apple, olive oil, salt and pepper. Toss well.

Add the juice from ¼ orange, add tomatoes, and toss well.

Grate zest over top and serve.

Glynis' Tip:

As you can see from the recipes, you can eat hearty and satisfying meals. When eating 2 meals a day, it's important to make them big enough to satisfy you and not leave you hungry. When I skip breakfast, do my exercise and then eat lunch, I make sure I eat plenty of protein. Fleur explained how important it is to keep protein levels up with my exercise regime. I will have an entire packet of either smoked salmon, sliced turkey or a tin of tuna and then add 2 boiled eggs as well. Plus lots of vegetables. When I haven't got much in my fridge, my fallback is always eggs. Scrambled with mushrooms (which count as protein) or a 3 egg omelette filled with whatever vegetables I have in my fridge. All followed by fruit and usually a cup of green tea. I can honestly say there are days I struggle to finish all that.

Footnotes

1. Peters A. et al. The Selfish Brain: competition for energy resources. *American Journal of Human Biology.* Vol 23, Issue 1 29-34. Feb 2011.
2. Sofer S. et al. Greater weight loss and hormonal changes after six months diet with carbohydrates eaten mostly at dinner. Obesity (Silver Spring) 19(10) 2006-14. October 2011.
3. Dazert E and Hall M.N. mTOR signalling in disease. *Current opinion in cell biology.* Vol 23, Issue 6 pp 744-755. December 2011.

Chapter Nine

Getting enough sleep and maintaining your circadian rhythm

Listen to your natural rhythm and get enough sleep

You have many different clock genes in your body, all regulated by a tiny nucleus in your brain, in the hypothalamus. The hypothalamus tends to be the master controller of your brain, as well as your body. It regulates your metabolism and controls your hunger and thirst. Maintaining a normal biorhythm is essential to the *In-Sync* programme as it will help you to burn fat and reach your ideal body composition. In other words, you will burn fat while you are asleep.

The first place to start to regulate your biological clock is by getting enough sleep! You should try to aim for around seven to eight hours per night depending on what you feel you personally need. A lot of studies have been done on the effects of sleep on our health and lifespan. Basically too much is as bad for your health as too little and both can disrupt your natural biorhythms and, therefore, your metabolism can wreak havoc on your appetite. What is more, researchers at medical school in Singapore showed that the less sleep older adults get, the faster their brains age. [1]

You should also avoid anything longer than a brief 'power nap' in the afternoon as this too may affect your circadian rhythm.

Glynis' Tip:

Amazing that you can burn fat while you sleep isn't it? But by the same token, if you don't sleep well on a regular basis, lack of sleep can make you gain weight. Yup, that's right, not only can drinking water regularly but incorrectly make you fat, so can sleep deprivation! It just goes to show how incredibly important it is to be In-Sync! Modern life and all the technology, processed foods, chemicals (this list could go on forever) keep us out of tune with ourselves, out of sync. But there is so much you can do to get yourself back on track and that is the very purpose of this book.

Sleep is a big issue for me. My entire adult life I have struggled with it. And I've tried everything. I've seen the negative effects on my life when I go through a phase of very poor sleep. Oh, how I envy those lucky people who fall asleep the minute their head hits the pillow.

However, I now have some very effective strategies that have helped me enormously. The single most effective thing has been eating The In-Sync Diet. *I eat a lot more protein now and that has made the biggest difference of all. I thought I was eating ample protein before but when Fleur took my measurements she found that with the amount of exercise I was doing, I needed quite a bit more protein. Finding myself then sleeping like a baby for the first time in years was a bonus I hadn't expected. The other thing is to be quite disciplined about the time I get into bed and turn out the light. I found that the later I leave it, the less well I sleep.*

Early Birds and Night Owls

Most of us tend to be early birds because our ancestors came from Africa. They developed a 'hunt by day, sleep at night' rhythm which enabled them to avoid being eaten by the lions and other predators that would sleep during the day. Being an 'early bird' suggests that you probably function better when you get up early in the morning and go to bed at a reasonable time at night. You may also prefer to do your physical activity, whenever possible, in the morning.

Some of our ancestors, however, would have been the 'night guards' in Africa which means a few of us may be more of a night owl than an early bird. If you feel you are a night bird, you may prefer to go to bed a little later and do more activities such as exercise at night. You may even suffer less from jet lag than your early bird counterparts. If you are a 'night owl' you should be conscious of getting enough sleep.

What is the melatonin connection?

Melatonin is a hormone which makes you feel sleepy. It is produced once daylight starts to fade so that you feel drowsy and ready to fall asleep. Once it is dawn melatonin production is switched off.

When the signals get disturbed

Nowadays instead of the evenings getting darker and darker they are getting lighter and lighter - and all because of artificial light. The result is less melatonin production which can interfere with your natural sleep-wake cycle.

Being mindful of avoiding any potential circadian rhythm disruptors such as exposure to light at night can go a long way towards ensuring you are producing sufficient melatonin. To help you, The In-Sync Diet has provided a checklist of actions you can take.

A checklist of actions to improve your sleep

Minimize or Avoid Stimulants

- Avoid alcohol (wine, beer and spirits) within 3 hours before bedtime.
- Avoid caffeine-containing beverages or foods after 2 pm.
- Avoid decongestant cold medicines at night.
- Some medications may have stimulating effects. Consult your pharmacist and doctor to determine whether any of them might be contributing to sleep problems.
- Complete any aerobic exercise at least three hours before bedtime.

Bedroom Air Quality

- Keep your bedroom air clean.
- Avoid toxic glues or other items producing an odour.
- If you see mould or have a musty smell in your bedroom, have it cleaned appropriately.
- Consider a saline spray before bed if your nose is blocked.

Night Time Tension and Anxiety

- Avoid anxiety proving activities close to bedtime:
- Avoid reading or watching news before going to bed.
- Avoid reading stimulating or exciting materials in bed.
- Avoid paying bills before bed.
- Avoid checking your financial reports or the stock market before bedtime.
- Avoid arguments before bedtime.
- Schedule difficult conversations well before bedtime.

Sleep Planning and Bedroom Preparation

- Schedule your sleep in if need be for 8 hours.
- Aim to go to bed no later than 11 pm during the week and wake up at the same time each morning to train your biological clock.
- Avoid getting into bed after midnight as often as possible as late-hour sleep may not be as helpful.
- Avoid later afternoon or evening naps.
- Avoid large meals or spicy foods before going to bed.
- Finish eating a couple of hours before bedtime.
- Avoid drinking too much water before bedtime.

Strategies to use with Trouble Falling Asleep or Staying Asleep

- Consider reading a good neutral book under low night light to help with falling asleep.
- Don't stay in bed more than 20 - 30 minutes to fall asleep. Leave your bedroom and go to another relaxing room or do a relaxation technique.
- If you wake up early because of the light, put a dark covering over your eyes.
- If you wake up early because of recurrent thoughts, try writing them in a journal.

Light, Noise, Temperature and Environmental Issues

- Turn down the light in the bathroom and in the rooms you are in fifteen minutes before going to bed.
- Decrease the light in your bedroom by using a dimmer or reading light.
- Use dark window shades or consider a set of dark eye shades or black covering for your eyes when trying to sleep or if you wake up too early because of the light.
- Decrease irritating noises in your space by closing windows or using ear plugs.

- Turn off or remove any appliances or clocks that make a noise.
- Make sure your sleeping area is the correct temperature - not too hot or too cold.
- Avoid sleeping near electric fields. Possible electrical fields include clock radios, computers, monitors and mobile phones. If you use your smartphone as an alarm clock, make sure you put it into aeroplane mode.

Getting rid of blue light

Blue wavelength light is harmful to circadian rhythm. It can suppress melatonin production more than ultra-violet light yet it can be emitted from electronic devices such as computer screens and TV screens, energy-efficient light bulbs, fluorescent light bulbs and LED lights.[2] One solution for those who have to work at night, for example, night shift workers who are more exposed to this type of light, is to use blue light blocking glasses.[3]

Shift workers are at especially high risk for circadian rhythm disruptions, because of their non-biorhythm friendly schedules. In a study by scientists from Quebec, nightshift workers wore blue light blocking glasses at or near the end of their overnight shifts for 4 weeks. At the end of study period, their overall sleep amounts increased, as did their sleep efficiency.[4]

Top Tip:

Blue light blocking glasses are also useful for breastfeeding mums to wear at night as quite often baby monitors will have a blue light.

Top Tip:

Chicken, turkey, salmon, asparagus and eggs are great sources of tryptophan. Tryptophan is a protein that is converted into serotonin - the neurotransmitter we attribute to feelings of wellbeing and happiness. Serotonin is converted to melatonin which we mentioned above as it regulates our sleep/wake cycle. In order to produce plenty of melatonin at night, make sure you eat plenty of tryptophan sources during the day.

Footnotes

1. Lo J.C. et al. Sleep duration and age-related changes in brain structure and cognitive performance. *Sleep* 37(7);1171-1178. 2014.
2. Czeisler C.A. Perspective: Casting light on sleep deficiency. *Nature* 497, 513. 23rd May 2013.

3. Burkhart K. and Phelps J.R. Amber lenses to block blue light and improve sleep. *Chronobiol Int* 8, 1602-12. December 2009.
4. Sasseville A. et al. Wearing blue-blockers in the morning could improve sleep of workers on a permanent night schedule: a pilot study. *Chronobiol Int* 26(5) 913-25. July 2009.

Chapter Ten

Getting Moving - The long slow workout

In Chapter Seven we made the case for doing short bursts of high-intensity exercise on an empty stomach which makes immediate changes to your body composition. Getting back to exercise or even starting an exercise regime for the first time can be daunting let alone doing it without having a bite to eat first. But actually your body can step up to the mark and make you better at burning fat. Exercise immediately switches on DNA to provide fuel to move even if you have never exercised before.[1]

In this chapter, we are going to introduce you to the long slow workout to add into your weekly activity routine alongside the high-intensity training you may be doing already. Endurance athletes such as marathon runners have to do it, to train their body to switch efficiently from burning sugar to burning fat.

Challenge that fat around the middle with a longer workout

From the time you begin to be physically active in your day, you will be burning fat but mainly you will be burning sugar. Your body really has to feel the need to use fat before you start to burn it efficiently. And quite often the fat that accumulates around the waist is the most stubborn and hangs around the longest. The way to get rid of stubborn fat is to challenge it with the 'long slow' workout! This is all about moving at a much slower pace for a longer period of time.

Moving at a slower pace for a longer period of time means that eventually you will have no option but to lose that tum! If your lifestyle has previously been quite sedentary or you have been used to eating six times (meals and snacks) per day, you may not be an efficient fat burner at the start. The long-slow workout is definitely for you!

Implementing the long slow/low-intensity workout:

- Start off by deciding whether you would like to run, walk, cycle, swim, stair climb - it could be absolutely anything!
- If you are new to exercise, then you should start off slowly, gradually increasing your time by five or ten minutes each week.
- Give yourself a five to ten minute gradual warm-up and slowly build the intensity.
- Over the next few weeks you can work towards exercising beyond forty-five minutes up to an hour which is the point at which your body's stores of sugar will dwindle and your body will need to make the switch to predominantly fat burning.
- If you are no stranger to exercise, you should aim to run at a low intensity i.e. sixty to seventy percent of your maximum heart rate for over an hour and preferably closer to two.
- Aim to do this workout, as with the high-intensity interval training sessions, on an empty stomach then feast on the foods on your programme.
- Stretch all your main muscle groups afterwards.

Top Tip: You increase your mitochondria through exercise

Mitochondria are tiny powerhouses inside your cells that supply you with most of your energy. They do this by burning the fat you have either eaten or stored. And, what is more, when you are exercising on an empty stomach they multiply so they can burn even more fat. Researchers at Harvard University believe that it may even be possible to slow or reverse the effects of ageing simply by stimulating mitochondrial activity through exercise and diet.[2] Each day when you wake up why not plan your activity for the day. This will depend on how you have slept and what you have done the day before. Always ask yourself the following questions:

How long am I going to exercise for?
How often will I be able to include movement in my day?
What kind of intensity will I be exercising at today?

Top Tip: Exercise outdoors for greater enjoyment

There is nothing like being in a spectacular environment outside to motivate you. When you feel that all is well with your world, exercise becomes a pleasure. This is partly as a result of increased visual stimulation and also produced by the endorphin 'high' you get. A review from The Peninsula College of Medicine and Dentistry found that exercising outside was linked to increased feelings of vitality, greater energy levels and mental wellbeing.[3] Even if you live in the city, you can benefit from being outdoors by seeking out the green spaces to do your training in.

Top Tip: Why not set yourself a long-term goal

Set a goal for, say, 6 or 12 months' time for a major physical challenge. It should be a big enough challenge to make you have to put some effort into it. Ideally, you should share this challenge with at least one other person to help keep you motivated. For example, if you are able, it could involve trekking, running or cycling 50 or 100 miles. If something like that is out of your reach, then choose another goal that you can strive for. Invite some friends along to do it with you or join a club.

Glynis' Tip:

Talking of a long slow workout, one of my favourite things to do on a Sunday is to go to the gym and get on the treadmill and bike and read all the Sunday papers. Most trainers would probably baulk at that, but I make sure I keep my walking and cycling speed at a good level. With lots to entertain me, I manage to do at least an hour and get to read the papers in peace!

With exercise, it's always good to do a variety of things and mix it up a bit. The body gets used to a routine quite quickly if you always do the same old thing. For this reason, I try and do 3 different types of exercise a week. This consists of:

- *Yoga (my current favourite being hot yoga)*
- *Weight training (working with weights in the gym)*
- *Cardiovascular (usually a mixture of cross trainer, stationary bike and walking on the treadmill).*

On a good week, time allowing, I will do each of these twice. I usually end up working out 4 - 6 times a week. Sometimes I'll take a class instead e.g. Zumba, pilates, etc. When I'm away, I'll switch to swimming, cycling, hiking or whatever is available where I am. And sometimes I'll decide I just need a week of doing nothing, which is absolutely fine if you regularly exercise. Otherwise, holidays are a great opportunity to do something different.

Footnotes

1. Barres R. et al. Acute exercise remodels promoter methylation in human skeletal muscle. Cell Met. 15(3), pp 405-411. March 7, 2012.
2. Sinha M. et al. Restoring systemic GDF11 level reverses age-related dysfunctions in mouse-skeletal muscle. Science 9; 344; pp 649-652. May 2014.
3. Thompson J. et al. Does participating in physical activity in outdoor natural environments have a greater effect on physical and mental wellbeing than physical activity indoors? A systemic review. Environ. Sci. Technol. 45(5) pp 1761-1772. February 3, 2011.

Chapter Eleven

Phase Four - Weeks Five and Six

Congratulations you are about to start the fourth phase of the programme. At this stage, you may want to get your scales out again to see how you are doing or you may be able to tell the difference simply by feeling how your clothes are fitting you. *Remember that you should be weighing your body fat and not your body weight; your total body water should also have increased.*

By now you should have successfully begun to implement a healthy diet and exercise regime into your daily life. You will also have reduced the frequency with which you eat by skipping the odd breakfast here and there. By doing this, you are having an impact on your health and wellbeing as well as your ability to burn fat.

Summary of Phases One to Three of The In-Sync Diet:

- Drink enough water i.e. drink plenty to quench your thirst when you feel that you might be thirsty and don't drink again until you are.
- Don't snack! What this means is don't have anything in between meals that will cause an insulin response i.e. anything with calories. The only thing you should have between meals is water/green tea/red bush tea without sugar or milk. This also goes for after dinner - once you have finished your evening meal, don't go back into the kitchen!
- Always eat protein at the same meal as your vegetables/fruit.
- Minimise starchy carbs i.e. root vegetables and have them with your evening meal (potatoes, pasta, bread, etc. are not included in The In-Sync Diet).
- Use healthy fats every day like extra virgin olive oil, coconut oil (to keep you fuelled for longer), omega-3 fats from oily fish and undamaged saturated fats from grass-fed meats.
- 'Eat a rainbow every day' to boost your phytonutrient intake - go for as much colour variety in your fruit and vegetable choices as you can.
- Add in some short bursts of movement/high-intensity movement before you eat your first meal

of the day as hunger should be the signal to move not to eat (see Chapter Seven).

- Eat one to three servings of fruit per day with meals only.
- At least once per week do a 'long slow workout' working up to a time period of at least an hour to teach your body to effectively fat burn because your muscles have used up their sugar stores and there is no other choice. This could be done outdoors.
- Eat only three meals per day but **on two to three days per week, eat only two**. This is probably easiest done by skipping breakfast and having a late brunch. This is called 'intermittent fasting' and has been shown to be a much more effective weight loss strategy than calorie control.

Instructions for Phase Four of The In-Sync Diet

In Phase Four, we want you to take the next step and remove breakfast from your morning routine completely. This will increase your chances of burning fat because your nervous system which controls this process is activated by exercise and a lack of food. You will remember from earlier chapters that you have energy systems in place that will mean that your muscles will be provided with fuel even though you have not eaten. By doing this you are not only increasing your fitness, but your vitality and longevity too.

Instruction One:

Skip breakfast and eat only two meals per day. This is, as before, more easily done by having a late brunch and an early evening meal.

Glynis' Tip:

Skipping breakfast is the best option as it's easier to have a long period of not eating when you're asleep! However, if it just doesn't fit in with your schedule, then it's ok to skip lunch instead. It's important to remember to do some exercise before dinner.

Instruction Two:

Be as physically active as you can before you have your first meal see Chapters Seven and Ten.

Instruction Three:

Aim to have half a plate of good quality protein (refer to Chapter Six) and the other half vegetables. The vegetables may be steamed, sautéed, roasted or eaten raw with a dressing.

Instruction Four:

Moderate alcohol consumption can be continued if you wish. Please note that it is better to have it with meals as any alcohol that is drunk in the gaps between meals may interrupt the fat-burning potential. It should ideally be wine or spirits to reduce your lectin load (See Chapter Six).

Glynis' Tip:

As before, I would advise staying off the alcohol to maximise benefits and results. (I am now officially more of a tyrant than Fleur!) However, I'm speaking from experience. There is just no way I could do this while having my wine every night. Before I knew it, I would be nibbling away on bowls of nuts telling myself they're on the ok list so not a problem. Trust me if you eat dinner and then continue with your wine afterwards while adding snacks, you will NOT lose weight.

If you are capable (unlike me) of having one glass with your dinner and that's it, then you have my admiration and will be fine.

Top Tip:

There may be days when you do not feel able to exist on two meals alone. Energy levels can be affected by age, stress levels, medication, pregnancy, what you last ate, when your menstrual period is due and your level of fitness. You are the best judge of how you are feeling on a particular day. If you are feeling not quite up to par but do not want to stray too far away from the programme, try having a handful of berries for breakfast. Otherwise have three meals per day until you are feeling able to move back to two.

How to look after your mitochondria

In Chapter Ten we introduced you to your mitochondria. These are the tiny powerhouses inside your cells where most of your energy comes from. This energy is vitally important for all sorts of functions your body has to do from fat burning and muscle contraction through to food digestion and hormone production. But sometimes your mitochondria are simply not up to the job and this can result in poor energy supply. When your mitochondria slow down, all the functions in your body slow down, including your ability to reach your weight loss goal. By following The In-Sync Diet, you have all the necessary tools to look after your mitochondria so that your energy levels are optimal. These include eating a healthy cleansing diet, exercising on empty, drinking sufficient water and getting enough good quality sleep.

Twelve Foods that provide extra support for your mitochondria

These twelve foods have been recommended by The Alliance for Natural Health International [2] to improve mitochondrial function.

1. **Coconut Oil**

    Coconut oil has been misunderstood because of its saturated fat content. In fact, the saturated fat it contains is an extremely healthy fat known as medium-chain triglycerides (MCT's).[11] MCT's are very easily digested and do not need bile salts to be broken down. They go straight to the liver where they can be used as a quick source of fuel. They are associated with better blood sugar balance, increased fat metabolism, better appetite control and enhanced cognitive function.

Serving ideas:

- Add a tablespoon to your favourite smoothie
- Mix with coconut cream and add to your coffee to make a coconut latte.

Use it to cook with as it has a reasonably high smoke point. This means that it can be heated to a fairly high temperature, 180 degrees Celsius approximately, before it starts to oxidise and become dangerous to health.

2. Avocado

Avocados are an excellent source of a healthy kind of fat known as monounsaturated fatty acids. Studies show that eating foods rich in monounsaturated fats (MUFAs) can improve blood cholesterol levels, which can decrease your risk of heart disease. Research also shows that MUFAs may benefit blood sugar control too.[3] They also contain potassium, vitamin E, B vitamins and fibre. Eat a few slices around three times per week to reap the benefits.

Serving ideas:

- Chop up a couple of slices and add to a vegetable soup.
- Mix with onions, tomatoes and fresh coriander for guacamole.

3. Spinach

Spinach is a great provider of lutein which makes it an important food for supporting healthy eyesight and preventing macular degeneration and cataracts. In addition to lutein, researchers have discovered at least thirteen different compounds in spinach that function as antioxidants and anti-cancer agents.[4]

Because it is capable of accumulating large amounts of pesticide residues, you should eat organically grown.

Serving idea:

- Lightly sauté with garlic and olive oil and top with some freshly squeezed lemon.

4. Pomegranate

Pomegranate has four different plant chemicals, that have beneficial effects. Of these, punicalagin is the most notable because of its superior antioxidant, antifungal and antibacterial properties. In fact, it has the most powerful antioxidant properties of all the fruits as well as important immune-supporting effects. It has even been known to help in the reversal of atherosclerotic plaques.[6]

Serving ideas:

- Sprinkle over a dish of lamb.
- Add to a spinach salad with walnuts, olive oil and balsamic vinegar.

5. Blueberries

Blueberries are an excellent source of flavonoids. Flavonoids are a type of plant chemical, with antioxidant qualities and many other health benefits. The antioxidant compounds are responsible for their blue/purple pigment. They are also a good source of vitamin C, fibre, and manganese, vitamin E and riboflavin. Researchers have also found that blueberries help protect the brain from oxidative stress and may help protect against neurological disorders such as Alzheimer's.[7] Please note that we have selected blueberries here but all berries (strawberries, raspberries, etc.) have the above health giving properties.

Serving idea:

- Add ½ cup of fresh or frozen berries to your favourite smoothie or pancake recipe.

6. Seaweed

Seaweed or sea vegetables are incredibly rich in minerals - they offer the broadest range of minerals of any food. In particular, they are a good source of iodine which is often lacking in our diets. Iodine is an important antioxidant as well as providing material to make thyroid hormones. They are an excellent source of calcium, sodium, folic acid, magnesium, potassium and iron. Various types of seaweed, arame, kelp and Nori, can be found in supermarkets, health food shops and Asian shops.

Serving ideas:

- Wrap your own sushi in Nori sheets.
- Make vegetarian rolls with Nori sheet and thinly sliced salad vegetables such as cucumber and avocado.
- Sprinkle kelp flakes over your salad or soup.

7. Almonds

Almonds are rich in monounsaturated fat which is associated with a reduced risk of heart disease. They also contain two vital brain nutrients, riboflavin and L-carnitine. These have been shown to increase brain activity, resulting in new neural pathways and a decreased occurrence of autism and Alzheimer's disease.[8] [9] They also contain vitamin E, which accounts for their antioxidant action and are a good source of magnesium and potassium.

8. Wild Alaskan Salmon

Wild Alaskan salmon is a great source of omega-3 fatty acids. Omega-3 fatty acids are important for the functioning of your brain and every cell in your body. They also provide the raw materials for an anti-inflammatory reaction and so play an important part in the healing process. It is the antioxidant astaxanthin that gives Alaskan salmon its vibrant red colour. Astaxanthin is a very powerful antioxidant that acts as an anti-inflammatory offering support for the heart and the brain.[12]

Wild salmon versus farmed salmon

The benefits of eating wild salmon are so much greater than eating farmed. Farmed salmon tends to have a thicker layer of fat due to the diet it has been fed. Wild salmon contains a wide range of nutrients because it has eaten a natural diet. In contrast, farmed salmon is fed on a diet of grain products such as corn and soy. Farmed salmon tends to be reared in pens near the sea where there may be a high number of pollutants such as pesticides and antibiotics.

9.   Unrefined Extra Virgin Olive Oil

Olive oil has multiple benefits for health. Research has shown that cholesterol particles that are made up of olive oil are less likely to become oxidised and to adhere to blood vessel walls. Olive oil consumption has been linked to better blood sugar control and lower triglycerides in the blood. Olive oil contains oleic acid which is an omega-9 fatty acid important for heart health. It is also made up of mixed tocopherols, which means it is a great source of vitamin E. It can help with weight loss because it has a chemical compound, hydroxytyrosol, which encourages the growth of new mitochondria and also their fat-burning potential.[13]

Serving idea:

- Olive oil has a fairly low smoke point which means it is not a great oil to cook with at anything above 148 degrees Celsius. Instead drizzle it over vegetables for extra flavour and add to your salad dressing.

10. Grass-fed Beef

Grass-fed beef comes from animals that have grazed on pasture all year round. Cows can cleverly convert grass into meat that is easy for you to digest. They are able to do this because they are ruminants. This means they have a stomach that represents a fermentation tank complete with resident bacteria to do the job. Grass feeding livestock improves the quality of the beef and makes it richer in omega-3 fatty acids, vitamin C, vitamin E and conjugated linoleic acid (CLA). CLA is a fat that reduces the risk of cancer, obesity, diabetes and heart disease.[14]

Recipe idea

Homemade grass-fed beef burgers - Serves four

600 grammes grass-fed minced beef
1 chopped onion
1 free range egg yolk whisked
1 tablespoon mixed herbs
A crushed clove of garlic.
4 tablespoons of desiccated coconut (optional)
Some melted coconut oil (optional)
Sea salt and pepper to taste

Mix all the ingredients above (apart from the coconut oil and desiccated coconut) in a bowl. Shape the mixture into burgers and roll both sides in desiccated coconut that has been sprinkled over a surface (optional). Brush with some melted coconut oil (optional). Place burgers on a tray and grill for fifteen minutes, turning once or more, until done as you prefer.

Serve with plenty of fresh mixed salad and half a baked sweet potato.

Are grass-fed and organic the same?

Organic meat is that which is hormone and antibiotic free. However, this is not the same as grass-fed because an organically reared animal will have been fed on organically grown grain rather than grass. They may also have spent their lives in feedlots rather than open pasture. In the same way, grass-fed does not mean organic as animals may have been reared on pasture that has been treated with pesticides and herbicides. If you want the best, opt for organic and grass-fed. You may want to befriend an honest butcher so that you know you are getting the genuine article.

11. Mango

Mangoes are incredibly beneficial to health. This is due to their high concentration of carotenoids, antioxidants and numerous other plant chemicals. Compounds include vitamin C and beneficial flavonoids that appear to be responsible for their anticancer effects.[15] Mangoes, like papaya, contain a number of enzymes which can improve digestion. For this reason, in tropical countries it is often used as a meat tenderizer. They are also a source of vitamin E, potassium and magnesium.

Serving ideas:

• Add to a rice salad with carrot, pepper and celery.

- Serve with shrimps and red pepper for a delicious shrimp salad.
- Toss them into a green salad to add a tangy twist.

12. Broccoli

Last but certainly not least we are going to feature broccoli which is a member of the cruciferous, or cabbage, family of vegetables. The cruciferous family include broccoli, cabbage, kale, cauliflower, pak choi, Brussel sprouts, etc. They are so beneficial to health that The In-Sync Diet recommends that you include a portion of cruciferous vegetables every day. Broccoli contains glucosinolates such as indole-3-carbinole and sulforaphane which demonstrate remarkable anticancer effects, particularly in breast cancer.[16] Other health-giving nutrients include vitamins K, C and A as well as folic acid, magnesium and potassium.

Serving ideas:

- Add broccoli florets and chopped stalks to salads and omelettes or use as crudités.
- Lightly steam for 9 - 12 minutes or sauté.
- Sauté broccoli florets in olive oil with pine nuts and garlic.

If you really want to maximise weight loss, stay off the starchy vegetables and make sure that you have plenty of all other vegetables. (Remember that if, at any time, things aren't moving in your bowels, vegetables will help!)

The thing that makes this diet so doable is that you can eat really good sized portions with delicious ingredients and then have the sweetness of fruit to satisfy any sugar cravings afterwards. The fact that avocados are not only allowed but encouraged, to my mind makes it all so much easier. An avocado is very satisfying and can be eaten in so many ways. Added to a salad, halved and eaten with a vinaigrette sauce (with maybe chopped veggies or shrimps on top), or made into guacamole with cruditee to dip in. Also, olive oil dressing makes a salad so delicious. It's the lack of fat that makes most diets so unsatisfying and depressing. Being allowed portions of healthy fats makes a world of difference.

I had presumed mangoes would not be allowed because they're so sweet but no, it turns out they're good in every way! Woohoo! Mango pieces with a handful of coconut chunks make a delicious desert.

And don't forget eggs! Far from being the cholesterol causing villains of myth, it turns out they are just about the perfect protein. Forget the egg white only omelettes

155

and always eat the whole egg. I get through probably a dozen eggs a week. I love them, have always loved them and have eaten them daily since childhood.

The other thing that I've newly rediscovered is mushrooms. However, they absorb everything from the soil in which they're grown so very important to stick to organic ones. They count as protein. I will often sauté sliced mushrooms in a bit of butter. Sounds wrong and unhealthy doesn't it? But no, this is a very healthy and nutritious option.

My American Brussel Sprout Salad:

I hate brussel sprouts! I've not eaten them since I was very young and was made to. However, when I was in California recently, I kept coming across brussel sprout salads. I thought it was beyond weird to have such a thing until I went to a friends' house and she served her version of it. It would've been rude not to so I tentatively had a mouthful and to my amazement loved it so much I went back for seconds….and then asked for the recipe. When I returned to England and made it at home, my son, who refuses all salads, did the same thing and now asks me to make it all the time.

1 ¾ lbs / 660g brussel sprouts
1 cup almonds well toasted
3 tablespoons finely grated Reggiano Parmigiano (as we

are still at the dairy free stage of the diet, you should leave this part out. When you get to the maintenance stage you could start adding it)
2 tablespoons finely chopped chives (save a little for garnishing)
1/3 cup / 75ml olive oil
2 tablespoons truffle oil (hard to find but I found an olive oil that has truffle oil in it)
2 tablespoons lemon juice
½ teaspoon salt
½ teaspoon freshly ground pepper
¾ cup of dried cranberries (dried fruit is high in sugar so not ideal. Could easily be left out or just add a small handful. Fleur says that the incredible nutritious goodness of the sprouts makes it ok to add just a few)

1. *Wash the sprouts and slice as thinly as possible*
2. *Make the dressing by mixing the olive and truffle oils, lemon juice, salt and pepper*
3. *Toss the sprouts, almonds, cranberries, cheese and chives together and then toss in the dressing.*
4. *Sprinkle on a few chives to garnish*

NB *Unless you live in California, this is essentially a winter salad as sprouts are normally only available then and it's always best to eat things that are in season.*

Footnotes

1. Myhill S. et al. Chronic fatigue syndrome and mitochondrial dysfunction. *Int. J.Clin Exp.Med.*2(1), 1-16, January 15, 2009.
2. Verkerk R. Build your energy reserve or age prematurely and die early. ANH-Intl feature 5 June 2013.
3. Cho M.J. et al. Flavonoid content and antioxidant capacity of spinach genotypes determined by high-performance liquid chromatography/mass spectrometry. *Journal of the Science of Food and Agriculture* Vol 88, Issue 6 pp 1099-1106. April 2008.
4. Paniagua J. et al. A MUFA-Rich diet improves postprandial glucose, lipid and GLP-1 responses in insulin-resistant subjects. *Journal of the American College of Nutrition.* Vol. 26, Issue 5, 2007.
5. Aviram M. et al. Pomegranate juice consumption reduces oxidative stress, atherogenic modifications to LDL, and platelet aggregation: studies in humans and in atherosclerotic apolipoprotein E-deficient mice. *Am J Clin Nutr* 2000;71(5):1062-76.
6. Ramassamy C. Emerging role of polyphenolic compounds in the treatment of neurodegenerative diseases: A review of their intracellular targets. *European Journal of Pharmacology* Volume 545, Issue 1, 1 September 2008 pages 51-84.
7. Rossignol D.A. and Bradstreet J.J. Evidence of mitochondrial dysfunction in autism and implications for treatment. *American Journal of Biochemistry and Biotechnology* Vol. 4, Issue 2, pp 208-217, 2008.
8. Butterfield D.A. et al. Nutritional approaches to combat oxidative stress in Alzheimer's disease. *The Journal of Nutritional Biochemistry* vol 13, issue 8 pp 444-461 August 2002.
9. Scholz-Ahrens K.E. et al. Prebiotics, Probiotics and Synbiotics affect mineral absorption, bone mineral content and bone structure. *The Journal of Nutrition* vol 137 no 3 8385-8465 March 2007.

10. Marten B et al. Medium-chain triglycerides. *International Dairy Journal* Vol 16, Issue 11, pp137401382, November 2006.

11. Rishton G.M. Natural products as a robust source of new drugs and drug leads: past successes and present day issues. *The American Journal of Cardiology* vol 101, issue 10, Supplement 22 May 2008.

12. Hao J et al. Hydroxytyrosol promotes mitochondrial biogenesis and mitochondrial function in 3T3-L1 adipocytes. *Journal of Nutritional Biochemistry* 2009.

13. Daley C.A. et al. A review of fatty acid profiles and antioxidant content in grass-fed and grain-fed beef. *Nutrition Journal* 9:10 2010.

14. Percival S et al. Neoplastic transformation of BALB/3T3 cells and cell cycle of HL-60 cells are inhibited by mango juice and mango juice extracts. *J. Nutr* vol 136 no 5 1300-1304 May 2006.

15. National Cancer Institute. Cruciferous vegetable and cancer prevention. 06/072012.

Chapter Twelve

Healthy Hormone Balance

Your hormones are the chemical messengers of your body. They allow your organs and tissues to communicate with one another on the subjects of digestion, growth, emotions and even behaviour. But not only that, they control every aspect of weight management from your metabolic rate to appetite, to where you store fat to whether you are suffering from uncontrollable cravings. Having a healthy hormone balance will help you to reach your weight loss goal and maintain it

Glynis' Tip:

If you are a man, you may want to look away until after the next few pages! However, keep with it after that because demon hormones affect us all!

How female hormones work

Whilst a woman is sexually mature, she will be producing oestrogen and progesterone from the ovaries in a cyclical rhythm to produce a mid-cycle ovulation. Ovulation is the point at which an egg is released from the ovaries to be made available for fertilisation by sperm. If no fertilisation occurs, then the lining of the womb is shed during menstruation. Production of these 'ovary' hormones will regularly change according to the stage of the cycle. But sometimes normal hormone production can be upset by lifestyle factors such as diet, exercise, lack of sleep and stress.[1]

What if your hormones are letting you down?

If you are suffering any of the following symptoms during your cycle, it may be a sign that your hormones are out-of-sync.

Symptoms of Pre-Menstrual Tension (PMT)

Physical	Psychological
Dizziness	Anxiety
Bloating and weight gain	Depression
Breast tenderness	Tension
Abdominal pain	Irritability
Headache	Aggression

The changeover at menopause

Even if your hormones have been regular all your life, they may start to become irregular when you approach menopause. Once you have reached menopause, your body does produce lesser amounts of sex hormones (oestrogen, progesterone and testosterone). But while menstruation stops, hormone production definitely still continues. Instead of these hormones coming from the ovaries, they come from other parts of the body such as your adrenal glands and fat tissue. As with PMS, a combination of poor diet, lack of exercise, bad sleep habits can all contribute to some of the familiar symptoms of menopause [1]:

Familiar symptoms of menopause

Increase in fat gain especially around the middle	Fluid retention - swollen ankles and feet
Skin is less elastic	Vaginal dryness
Hot flushes	Loss of bone density
Loss of muscle mass	Lack of self-respect
Increase in fat gain especially around the middle	Fluid retention - swollen ankles and feet

But it does not have to be this way - menopause is not a pathological condition! Studies show that Asian women are symptom-free during their menopause whilst living in their native country. It is only when they move to the West and change their lifestyle that they succumb to the negative symptoms of menopause (above).[2] The following tips will help to achieve a healthy hormone balance whilst you are on The In-Sync Diet and beyond.

Tip One: Your hormones will be affected by your sleep/wake rhythm

In Chapter Nine, The In-Sync Diet stressed the importance of getting enough sleep to regulate your biological clock. Because the hormones oestrogen and progesterone are produced in a cyclical rhythm, they will be affected by any disruptions in your sleep/wake cycle.[3] These disruptions can lead to the symptoms of PMT and menopause shown earlier. Addressing your biorhythms by getting enough sleep and exercising on an empty stomach as well as reducing the number of times you eat can have tremendous benefits.

Tip Two: Good hormone control depends on balanced insulin levels

Insulin is a hormone that regulates your metabolism of sugars and fat. It does this by instructing your muscles and fat cells to take up sugar from the bloodstream once you have eaten. When you have had a meal that is particularly high in starchy carbs such as pasta, potatoes, cakes and sweets, then a lot of insulin is required to get rid of it. If you have been eating a diet that is rich in these high-calorie foods on a regular basis, chances are that your blood sugar levels are imbalanced and your hormones are out-of-sync.[4] All the foods that we have recommended on The In-Sync Diet will help you to balance your blood sugar levels and your hormones too.

Tip Three: Look after your liver

You began The In-Sync Diet with a two-day cleanse. This was to prepare your body to reach your weight loss goal. The problem is that we live in a modern environment that is full of chemicals. And these chemicals are known as 'obesogens' because they are capable of overloading your mitochondria so that you are no longer able to metabolise effectively and burn fat.[5] Because they go to the liver to be got rid of alongside any excess hormones, your liver can suffer too!

If your hormones are still out-of-kilter by this stage of the programme, you may need to implement some of the following to further reduce your 'toxic load'. A toxin can be anything that hampers the normal functioning of the body. By reducing your toxic load, you are re-laying strong foundations from which to maintain a toned body shape, stay in good health and have bundles of energy.

Here are some ideas you should start to implement:

- Aim to ensure that as much of your food as possible is organic. An additional benefit is that organic food contains higher levels of nutrients.
- If your digestion allows, include plenty of raw plant food into your diet to avoid the harmful effects of cooking foods at high temperatures.

- Limit your exposure to electromagnetic radiation by using a headset with your mobile phone and not actually putting your laptop on your lap. At night put your mobile phone in aeroplane mode and turn off your router.
- Use plant-based beauty and cleaning products and fluoride-free toothpaste. Keep your home well ventilated if you are going to be exposed to chemicals from new furniture, carpets or paint.
- Drink water from glass bottles rather than plastic.
- Have a sauna every week - see Chapter Five.
- Exercise regularly.
- Moderate your alcohol intake to small amounts during meals only.
- Get some fresh air on a daily basis.

By doing this, you will be reducing your exposure to xenoestrogens which are environmental chemicals that mimic female oestrogens.[6] These synthetic chemicals can really mess up your hormone balance.

Tip Four: Reduce your stress

Stress is a completely normal physiological response to a situation that you perceive as 'dangerous'. When you feel under threat, your body responds by releasing stress hormones such as adrenaline and cortisol that prepare you to deal with the situation. Your heart starts to beat faster, your muscles contract, ready for action, your blood pressure rises and your senses become more alert. The problem comes when you have been feeling under pressure for a long period of time as this can mean the constant release of stress hormones. This is not only draining on your energy levels, but it will affect your sex hormone production too. In the next chapter, you will learn some meditation techniques to help you put your stress to one side.

Tip Five: Try a forest bath!

Participating in 'forest bathing' trips is recommended as part of a healthy lifestyle in Japan.[7] A forest bathing trip (Shinrin-yoku) will allow you to soak in the tranquil atmosphere, admire the beautiful scenery and take in the clean, fresh air. But not only that, it offers a natural kind of aromatherapy - breathing in the organic compounds alpha-pinene and limonene may reduce stress and boost your immune system. You do not need to go to Japan to get the benefits - just walk around your nearest forest or even a park will do!

Glynis' Tip:

So not only do we have hormones to deal with but now "obesogens"??? Are you kidding me? Even the name is offensive!

At this point, I'm feeling ever so slightly smug though because I decided to eat as organically as possible as far back as the 1980's. No mean feat I can assure you. There was very little to be had and all my friends thought I was slightly unhinged. No one could really see the point of it back then. It was a very lonely arduous path. There was just me, Prince Charles and a smattering of lentil eating vegetarian hippies!

I was in absolute seventh heaven when I moved to California in 1990 and discovered a whole organic supermarket called Mrs. Gooches (bought out a few years later by the juggernaut that is now Whole Foods). I returned to the UK a few years later with absolute dread as to what I was going to find. With good reason, it turned out. However, now we are spoilt for choice and every single market will have at least some organic produce.

I love the sound of a forest bath, which is in fact just as tranquil as walking in a heavily wooded place. I say just, but actually this really is a wonderful thing to do. There's a place that I go to about once a year and do just that. I always feel so rejuvenated afterwards and just wish I could go more often. I'm such a city girl but actually find myself craving nature at times. I also love being near the sea. There's something about it that is incredibly soothing and meditative.

Footnotes

1. Ruiz-Nunez B, Pruimboom L et al. Lifestyle and nutritional imbalances associated with Western diseases: causes and consequences of chronic systemic low-grade inflammation in an evolutionary context. *The Journal of Nutritional Biochemistry,* vol 24, Issue 7, pages 1103-1201. July 2013.
2. Lock M. and Kaufert P. Menopause, local biologies and cultures of ageing. Am. J. Hum. Biol. 494-509. 2001.
3. Boden M.J et al. Circadian rhythms and reproduction. Reproduction 132 379-392. Sept 1 20006.
4. Milewicz A. and Jedrzejdlo D. Premenstrual syndromes from aetiology to treatment. *Maturitas,* Volume 55 Supplement 1, pages 547-554 November 2006.
5. Grun F and Blumbert B. Environmental obesogens. *Endocrinology* Volume 147, Issue 6, July 1, 2013.
6. Ryder M. Gender-bending xenoestrogens: if they're a problem for fish they could be a problem for you. *The Alliance for Natural Health* 24 September 2014.
7. Li Q et al. Forest bathing enhances natural killer cell activity in males and females. *Int J Immunopathol Pharmacol*: 2007,20(2 Suppl 2):3-8.

Chapter Thirteen

Part One: Training Your Large Muscle Groups

From the beginning of the programme, The In-Sync Diet has stressed the importance of keeping hold of your muscle mass whilst burning fat. This will really work in your favour because muscle is responsible for burning fat. Basically the more muscle you have on your body, the more fat you will burn.

By focusing on exercising the large muscle groups, (see examples on the next pages) at least twice per week, you will ensure that you will be burning fat. You will also be improving the density and strength of your muscles, which is associated with healthy ageing.[1] Rest assured you will not be 'bulking up' but working towards getting the lean toned look you are striving for.

Weight bearing exercise for post-menopausal women

For those of you who are at the early stages of menopause (peri-menopausal) or have gone through menopause, it is really important that you train your large muscle groups. This is because, with the decline of oestrogen levels associated with menopause, you may be more susceptible to muscle atrophy or general weakening of muscle.[2] The problem is that with a reduction of muscle quality, muscle tissue will be replaced with fat tissue. By introducing a regular routine of building up muscle strength, you will be helping to prevent any changes in muscle metabolism that can result in the loss of muscle strength.

Training with weights will also help to slow down age-related bone loss. Studies show that weight-bearing exercise, along with bone supporting nutrients, can maintain bone density in women at the early post-menopausal stage and help prevent osteoporosis.[3] Because bones are naturally broken down and rebuilt in tandem with your biological clock, it is also important that you get enough good quality sleep - please see Chapter Nine - Getting Enough Sleep.

Top Tip: Weight training/training large muscle groups will increase your fast twitch muscle fibres

Fast twitch muscle fibres produce the quick, powerful bursts of speed that can be seen in sprinters and weight lifters. They allow for rapid, powerful movement, but they are quick to tire. In contrast, 'slow twitch' muscle fibres fire more slowly and so are common to endurance athletes. Fast twitch fibres are also more likely to weaken than slow twitch muscle fibres as we age.

How to get started at home

Lunges:

- Keep your upper body straight, with your shoulders back and relaxed and chin up (pick a point to stare at in front of you so you don't keep looking down). Always engage your core.
- Step forward with one leg, lowering your hips until both knees are bent at about a 90-degree angle. Make sure your front knee is directly above your ankle, not pushed out too far and make sure your other knee doesn't touch the floor.
- Keep the weight on your heels as you push back up to the starting position.

- Repeat these twelve times to complete one set. Repeat each set six times.

Tricep dips:

- Position your hands shoulder-width apart on a secured bench or stable chair.
- Slide your bottom off the front of the bench with your legs extended out in front of you.
- Straighten your arms maintaining a little bend in your elbows to keep the tension on your triceps and away from your elbow joints.
- Slowly bend your elbows to lower your body towards the floor until your elbows are at about a 90-degree angle. Be sure to keep your back close to the bench.
- Once you reach the bottom of the movement, press down into the bench to straighten your elbows, returning to the starting position. This completes one repetition.
- Keep your shoulders down as you lower and raise your body. You can bend your legs to modify this exercise.
- Repeat these eight times to complete one set. Repeat each set ten times.

Bicep Curls:

You can use a pair of dumbbells for this or two items of equal weight that you can hold easily in your hand.

- Hold a dumbbell in each hand and stand with your feet as wide apart as your hips.
- Let your arms hang down at your sides with your palms facing forward.
- Pull your abdominals in, stand tall and keep your knees slightly bent.
- Curl both arms upward until they are in front of your shoulders.
- Slowly lower the dumbbells back down.
- Repeat these four times to a complete a set. Repeat each set twelve times.

Glynis' Tip:

Even though I love exercise and have always been very active, it does not mean I'm not a wimp. And even though I'm motivated to get to the gym, it doesn't mean I'm not a bit lazy. The thing is, I'll get there and then just not push myself very much. I have loads of excuses for this. I'm a bit tired, I'm not really in the mood, I don't want to hurt myself with heavy weights or (my favourite) I'm in a bit of a hurry!

People like me really need the help of a trainer. I recently put myself into a self-imposed boot camp under the supervision of Fleur for nutrition and a personal trainer to maximise my workouts. I explained to my trainer that I have bad knees and a bad back but did he care? He made me do the very things I thought would make these conditions worse. He made me lunge, squat and bend those knees to a degree I thought would make them actually snap in two. I was horrified. He then gave me very heavy weights. I've never been known for my brute strength! He made me do dead lifts which are basically standing with legs apart, knees bent, holding onto a metal rod with heavy weights attached. You then straighten your legs as you lift this massive weight. This, for a person with a bad back???

But here's the extraordinary thing, my knees and my back not only didn't suffer, they massively improved. There is no doubt that I'm stronger and fitter and more mobile with less pain in these joints.

Trainers can be expensive so a good option is to just book 1 or 2 sessions to get yourself set up and working out properly with those heavy weights. In fact, if you join a gym, you will usually be offered a session with one of their in-house trainers. Check in and do another session with the trainer when funds allow.

Footnotes

1. Asikainen TM et al. Exercise for Health for early post-menopausal women. *Sports Medicine.* Volume 34, Issue 11 pp 753-778. September 20014.
2. Lee C.E. et al. The role of hormones, cytokines and heat shock proteins during age-related muscle loss. *Clinical Nutrition.* Volume 26, Issue 5, Pages 524-534. October 2007.
3. Engelke K. et al. Exercise maintains bone density at spine and hip. *Osteoporosis Int.* Volume 17, Issue 1 pp 153-142. January 2006.

Chapter Thirteen

Part Two: Yoga for stress relief and fat loss

There are many types of yoga practices but typically it combines stretching exercises and poses with deep breathing and meditation. Yoga will stretch and tone your muscles and keep your spine and joints flexible. It is accompanied by deep breathing which is believed will provide more oxygenated blood to your brain. It involves a sequence of moves or poses that are maintained for a number of breaths depending on the type of yoga being taught, for example, Hatha, Ashtanga, Anasara, Iyengar or Bikram.

Benefits beyond flexibility

The power of yoga is such that it has an incredible impact on your body, but it also has an equally as powerful effect on your mind. Alongside decreasing your heart rate and blood pressure and increasing your muscle strength [1], yoga has the capacity to reduce stress and anxiety. [2] It also improves the quantity and quality of your sleep [3] which will help you to achieve hormone balance and lose fat too. In one study, after twelve weeks of yoga a group of people had all reduced the amount they ate as well as the speed at which they ate.[4] In another study, participants on a six-day yoga programme showed decreased body mass, reduced waist and hip circumference and had lost fat mass too.[5]

Glynis' Tip:

I started doing yoga nearly 30 years ago and it's very much a part of my life. I began when I was filming a TV series (Dempsey & Makepeace in case you're interested), working very long hours with quite a bit of stress. I may have been young at the time but it was immediately apparent to me how calming and beneficial yoga was.

I think it's wonderful for anyone, of any gender and of any age. However, as you age, I think it's one of the most effective things you can do to keep supple, toned, calm and youthful.

In fact, when I began to digress from my acting path into the world of health, the first thing I did was make an Anti-Ageing Yoga DVD.

There are many ways to start yoga. You could get a simple easy to follow DVD or you could go to a class. There are so many yoga classes, so many different types of yoga, that you are really spoilt for choice. I think a simple Hatha yoga style is a good place to start, but it really doesn't matter. If you do a class and don't like it, try another.

Yoga is not a competitive sport. You can easily have people at many different levels in the same class doing the same postures, all at their own level.

I've recently been doing hot yoga classes and I love them. Hot yoga is different to Bikram, which is also hugely popular. However, hot yoga is less hot than Bikram and it's more of a flowing class going from one pose to another. In Bikram, postures will be held for much longer. Each to their own.

The great thing about yoga is you can do it anywhere and anyhow. It's wonderful to do self-practice and go through some postures on your own once you are familiar with it.

Breathing is a very important part of yoga. You breathe deeply through your nose as you go in and out of postures. Most of us don't breathe properly (you'd think it would come naturally, wouldn't you?) and this is a wonderful way of getting the system properly oxygenated. It also has a calming effect on the nervous system.

I've explored many facets of yoga, including meditation. This too is hugely beneficial, particularly for stress and for problem solving. Meditating is a discipline. You need to commit to finding the time on a daily basis. I go through phases of this but when I do, there is no doubt I'm better for it. There's much scientific evidence to support its benefit, so well worth considering.

Here is a simple guided meditation for you to follow written by my husband, Michael Brandon. Besides being an actor, he has taught meditation for many years. He's taught in some of the toughest prisons in both the U.S. and the U.K. as well as The Priory rehab centre. I would suggest recording it, speaking very, very slowly, and then play it back while you lie down on your back listening to the instructions.

Visual Meditation

Start by lying flat on your back on the floor or on a mat. Begin by taking a deep breath and slowly exhaling. After three deep breaths, starting at your toes, imagine that they are filling with a warm golden oil.

Allow this warm golden oil to fill each foot, then the arches, the instep, then the heels and imagine the warm golden oil moving up your ankles to your calves and shins to knees and so on. No rushing, take the natural time it takes to allow this golden oil with its healing warmth to remove any tension or pain it comes across.

Bring the oil up into the thighs and into the buttocks and groin. Then let the oil fill your stomach, and move up the spine of your back. The oils' warmth healing and relaxing every part it touches. Now let it fill the chest and ribcage and as the oil surrounds your heart it glows with a golden hue. See the golden glow around your heart? Bring the oil up towards the neck and let it flow down into your arms to your elbows and to your hands. Feel the warm oil right to your finger tips. Slowly move back up your arms and into your shoulders removing all the tension and tightness as it moves up your neck into your head. Filling your skull, your facial bones, your ears, your lips, teeth and removing the tension around your eyes. Finally, let it fill your brain, all the way to the hair follicles on your head. Relaxing and calming your whole body. Breathe deep and let it all go. Like you're sinking into the floor. Just breathe.

You are now relaxed and are ready to meditate. Just lie there and go with it. Instead of letting your mind go all over the place, give it a focus; an action that occupies it so it leaves you in peace, like imagining a candle flame in the golden centre of your heart. This flame is steady and can't be blown out. Let the mind focus on the flame. As you focus on the flame, thoughts will still come and you can watch your thoughts but do not get involved with them.

Imagine your thoughts are like clouds in the sky floating by; you watch them blow across the sky of your mind. Just don't go with them. It happens with practice and soon a certain kind of detachment allows the mind to relax and be at peace. A clear sky becomes a calm mind.

Breathe and allow your mind to go deeper inside. Gently, like a fish swimming deeper into a beautiful sea without effort, let your mind go deeper within. This inner focus takes you to a calming place within yourself, the mountain top or the sea bottom within.

Here you can be still. Rejuvenate and leave all your problems or in fact find solutions to them, move on from them or see them not as problems. From detachment we still the frantic ramblings of the mind. When you breathe, you bring life to the cells of your body and in meditation you bring healing to your entire existence.

When you are ready, bring your awareness back to your body and the room. Take a deep breath and exhale...

Footnotes

1. Bijilani RL et al. A brief but comprehensive lifestyle education programme based on yoga reduces risk factors for cardiovascular disease and diabetes mellitus. *The Journal of Alternative and Complementary Medicine* 11(2): pp 267-274. April 2005
2. Smith C et al. A randomised comparative trial of yoga and relaxation to reduce stress and anxiety. *Complimentary Therapies in Medicine.* Volume 15, Issue 2, pp77-83, June 2007.

3. Chen K. M. et al. Sleep quality, depression state and health status of older adults after silver yoga exercises. *International Journal of Nursing Studies.* Volume 46, Issue 2, pp 154-163, February 2007.

4. Raju P.S. et al. Influence of intensive yoga training on physiological changes to six women: a case report. *The Journal of Alternate and Complementary Medicine.* Volume 3, Issue 3, September 2nd, 2007.

5. Telles S. et al. Short term health impact of yoga and diet change programme on obesity. *Med Sci. Monit.* (16) CR35-40, January 2010.

Chapter Fourteen

Final Phase - Weeks seven and eight

Congratulations you are about to start the final phase of the programme. At this stage, you may want to check in with yourself to see whether you are still drinking enough water. It is easy to slip back into old habits, especially where water is concerned. Again, if you are measuring your progress you might want to step onto the scales to make sure you are losing fat mass and not lean tissue. If you feel you are losing lean tissue, then you should increase your protein at meals and ensure you are doing some weight bearing exercises as in Chapter Thirteen - Part One.

Summary of Phases One to Phase Four of The In-Sync Diet:

- Drink enough water i.e. drink plenty to quench your thirst when you feel that you might be thirsty and don't drink again until you are.

- Don't snack! What this means is, don't have anything in between meals that will cause an insulin response i.e. anything with calories. The only thing you should have between meals is water/green tea/red bush tea without sugar or milk. This also goes for after dinner - once you have finished your evening meal, don't go back into the kitchen!

- Always eat protein at the same meal as your vegetables/fruit.

- Minimise starchy carbs e.g. root vegetables and if you chose to eat them, have them at night (potatoes, pasta, bread, etc. are not included in The In-Sync Diet).

- Use healthy fats every day like extra virgin olive oil, coconut oil (to keep you fuelled for longer), omega-3 fats from oily fish and undamaged saturated fats from grass-fed meats.

- 'Eat a rainbow every day' to boost your phytonutrient intake - go for as much colour variety in your fruit and vegetable choices as you can.

- Add in some short bursts of movement/high-intensity movement before you eat your first meal of the day, as hunger should be the signal to move not to eat (see Chapter Seven).

- Eat one to three servings of fruit per day with meals only.

- At least once per week do a 'long slow workout' working up to a time period of at least an hour to teach your body to effectively fat burn because your muscles have used up their sugar stores and there is no other choice.

- Remove breakfast from your morning routine completely. This will increase your chances of burning fat because your nervous system, which controls this process, is activated by exercise and a lack of food.
- Add in a couple of sessions per week of weight bearing exercise to train the large muscle groups in your body. This will not only increase your lean muscle, which is advantageous, particularly as we age, it will also improve bone density.
- Consider yoga if you haven't done already, as a weight management tool as well as an incredible way of regulating levels of stress and anxiety.

Instructions for The Final Phase of The In-Sync Diet

In The Final Phase, we want to introduce you to a 'luxury' meal! This is an opportunity for you to go 'freestyle'. Once per week you can enjoy your favourite meal without having to think whether it is allowed in *The In-Sync* programme or not. It can be one course, two courses or even three if you wish. And don't worry, in the grand scheme of things it will not affect your weight loss goals. All we ask is that you follow theses instructions.

Instruction One:

Your 'luxury' meal should only happen once per week. This will ensure you are still keeping your lectin load low and not compromising weight loss.

Instruction Two:

Your 'luxury' meal should include protein - preferably in every course! In the case of dessert, you could have cream or nuts or even cake!

Instruction Three:

You should drink a couple of glasses of water before and after your 'luxury' meal.

Glynis' Tip:

Ok, how exciting is this? Yes, that's right! You can eat anything...ANYTHING...you want...for one meal a week. When Fleur added this to my regime, I couldn't believe it. I was scared it would ruin my diet...make me put on weight...sully my incredibly (in my mind anyway) pure body! But on the contrary, it's really important to do this as it gives your metabolism a kick start.

And wow did it feel good. Mind you, I was so full and could really feel the effects the next day so was quite happy to get back to The In-Sync Diet.

Do remember in all your excitement to follow the instructions above regarding the protein and water though.

Why we comfort eat

The In-Sync Diet has encouraged you to move before you eat. Hunger should be a signal to go out and find food rather than eating before you go out. In our evolutionary past hunger would have been a stress signal to warn us to find food otherwise we would not survive! Finding food would have stopped that stress response and we could have sat and enjoyed our quarry.

Nowadays we tend to suffer from chronic stress i.e. there is constant pressure - the mortgage needs to be paid, the bills mount up, work demands are huge, the emails keep coming and so on. It is, therefore, perfectly natural that we should take comfort in food because that has an evolutionary history of being able to switch off the pressure temporarily. And not only that, we are having to fuel those feelings of constant stress because they are hugely energy consuming.

The brain, as we have mentioned previously, is the most

energy demanding organ of all. It represents such a small part of our body weight and yet it can consume up to two thirds of all the circulating, glucose, energy in the body.[1] The brain is provided for by the breakdown of protein, fat and carbohydrate into glucose. The problem is if we rely on eating sugar and refined carbohydrate foods every day or several times a day, the whole energy balance gets disturbed and we can suffer carbohydrate cravings.

Don't be tempted to go down the artificial sweetener route either. It is now official, see Chapter Six, that the regular consumption of artificial sweeteners will make you fat! [2] As long as you are using the many products that contain saccharin, aspartate, stevia, sorbitol and xylitol you will always feel the need to eat.

Your body can cope with having the occasional sugary foods, just not on a daily basis. The brain definitely loves a bit of sugar! And if you eat your sugar alongside your protein and fat the sugar will not have such a detrimental effect on your blood sugar levels. This can be done by having the 'luxury' meal and finishing it off with a dessert, you are a lot less likely to suffer from unstable blood sugar levels and food cravings afterwards.

When that 'feeling full' feeling does not come any more

The reason you feel full after a meal is all down to a hormone called leptin. Leptin is actually produced by the fat around our middle and is called a hormone because it sends messages to the rest of the body. It regulates appetite or more specifically satiety by sending a message to your brain to say that there is enough stored energy (in fat) and you do not need to eat any more at that moment. The brain needs this messaging system to make sure that the rest of the body does not run out of supplies to keep it functioning.[1]

Again moving before you eat is important here. If you eat before you are actually hungry, for example because your lunch-break at work is at a particular time, you will upset this messaging system. Not feeling hungry means that your storage centres are still full and leptin will not work as efficiently for you if you do eat. Satiety signals may not reach the brain and your fat tissue may respond by producing more and more leptin.

Over the course of time, this state of play can become far too much for your brain and eventually it will refuse to accept any more messages. The result of this could be that you do not know when to stop eating and you keep on putting on weight. The irony is that although you may have plenty of stored energy (fat) you cannot access it and so you feel too tired to move. This is known as leptin resistance. So how do you fine-tune this messaging system again?

The in-Sync Solutions

- Exercise, exercise, exercise! When you exercise, you form new mitochondria and these are the power houses of your cells where you burn the fat.
- Follow the food recommendations on The In-Sync Diet for moderate protein consumption with healthy fat and low carbohydrate from vegetables and fruit.
- If you are not hungry skip another meal, it does not only have to be breakfast!
- Move before you eat.

Top Tip: Dark chocolate can hit the spot instead of a sugary fix

The darker the chocolate, the less sugar it contains and the more beneficial to health. It has been suggested that regular sugar consumption is as addictive as regular cocaine consumption.[3] Certainly sugar prolongs the action of ghrelin which is a hormone produced in the stomach that tells us we need to eat. It also reduces the ability of leptin to inform the brain we have eaten enough. And it decreases our ability to enjoy our food as it suppresses the feeling of euphoria we can get from dopamine so we need to eat more and more each time to get our hit.[4]

Chocolate has been called a stimulant, relaxant, anti-depressant and even an aphrodisiac! But a study has shown that these effects may not be long-lasting particularly if we use chocolate as a tool for comfort eating or to satisfy cravings.[5]

The darker variety is so beneficial to health, however, that we can fit chocolate consumption in somewhere without feeling guilty about it. Studies show that it can lower blood pressure and reduce the likelihood of cardiovascular disease [6] and make our blood sugar levels more stable.[7] It is high in minerals such as magnesium and manganese as well as protein and healthy fats.

Because of the protein and fat content, it does have the ability to satisfy the appetite if eaten **in moderation**. Try melting a couple of squares on your tongue before your luxury meal to keep your appetite in check. Or enjoy it after a luxury meal to complete your palate.

This chapter just gets better and better doesn't it? I knew I was right about chocolate and have had a lifetime of testing it out! I made a conscious effort to move from the milk to the dark. Ok, I know that milk chocolate is yummy, but there is now a huge variety of really delicious dark chocolates. My favourites are with added sea salt, lavender, geranium and nuts. And yes I've really found all those. You do have to make sure though that whatever is added to the chocolate, hasn't also added a load of sugar and remember the darker the chocolate, the less sugar and the better for you it is.

In this final stage of the diet, only eat chocolate with your luxury meal. When you're on to the maintenance stage, you can add a small amount after a meal.

Gluten-free baking recipes:

These are included for those of you who prefer to stay gluten-free during your luxury meal or as an occasional treat when on the maintenance programme.

Beetroot and Banana Cake

3 ripe bananas
100g raw beetroot diced
150g coconut oil
4 large organic eggs
3 tablespoon (raw local) honey
1 heaped teaspoon bicarbonate of soda
100g coconut flour

Blend all wet ingredients until smooth (ideally use a high-speed blender or food processor).

Add in dry ingredients and blend well. You will have produced an amazingly lush red coloured mixture.

Line an ovenproof tin with parchment paper and add the mixture.

Cook at 180°C for 45-50 minutes until firm to touch and magic has turned your cake brown.

Chestnut Pancakes

125g chestnut flour
1 teaspoon ground cinnamon
1 teaspoon bicarbonate of soda
3 large organic eggs
500ml coconut milk or water
Handful of kale (if blending with high-speed blender)
Coconut oil

Blend all ingredients together until smooth.

Heat a teaspoon of coconut oil in a frying pan.

Add approximately tablespoon of mixture to form a drop scone sized pancake. Repeat to fill the pan.

Cook on medium heat for a minute or so on each side.

Serve with berries and natural yoghurt.

Pear and Chocolate Pudding

6 eggs
75g coconut oil
75g (grass-fed) organic unsalted butter
60g coconut sugar
2 tablespoon (raw local) honey
1teaspoon ground cinnamon
1 heaped teaspoon bicarbonate of soda
150ml coconut milk or water
2 teaspoon vanilla essence
60g coconut flour
60g raw cacao powder
3 pears sliced or diced

Mix together dry ingredients in a bowl. Blend wet ingredients (preferably in a high-speed blender or food processor) until smooth.

Add dry ingredients and blend well.

Butter the inside of a large shallow glass ovenproof dish. Add the pear and the pudding mixture.

Cook in a heated oven at 180°C for 35-40 minutes until risen and firm to touch.

Serve warm with natural yoghurt.

Footnotes

1. Peters A et al. The selfish brain: competition for energy resources. *Neurosci* (2) 143-80, April 20004.

2. Feijo F. de M. et al. Saccharin and aspartame, compared with sucrose, induce greater weight gain in adult Wistar rats at similar total caloric intake levels. *Appetite* 60(1) 203-7. January 2013.

3. Lenoir M. et al. Intense sweetness surpasses cocaine reward. DOI: 10.1371/journal.pone.000069. August 2007.

4. Lustig R.H. Sugar: The Bitter Truth. University of California Television (UCTV) Youtube July 20, 2009.

5. Parker G et al. Mood states of chocolate. *Journal of Affective Disorders* 92, 149-159, 2006.

6. Hooper L. et al. Effects of chocolate, cocoa and flavan-3-ols on cardiovascular health: a systematic review and meta-analysis of randomised trials. *Am J Clin Nutr* Vol 95, no 3, pp 740-751, March 2012.

7. Grassi D. et al. Short-term administration of dark chocolate is followed by a significant increase in insulin sensitivity and a decrease in blood pressure in healthy persons. *Am J Clin Nutr* Vol 81 No 3 611-14, March 2005.

Chapter Fifteen

Bring the brown fat back!

Have you ever known a baby to shiver with cold? The answer is probably not because babies are born into the world with a large supply of brown fat. Brown fat is so called because it has a large blood supply and plenty of fat burning iron-containing mitochondria that give it its colour. Unlike white fat which stores excess calories in unwanted places around our body, 'good' brown fat generates heat for us by burning excess calories. This is a process known as thermogenesis and is essential for our ability to cope with different temperatures particularly the cold.

Getting out of our thermal comfort zone

By hanging on to 'good' brown fat, we more easily adapt to cold temperatures which make us burn calories to produce heat at the same time! The problem is that nowadays we do not suffer cold lightly. We spend more time indoors with central heating that keeps our environment at a constantly ambient temperature.

Under floor heating, draught excluders, door seals, insulation and double glazing all ensure that as long as we are indoors, no cold will get to us. A group of researchers have suggested that by remaining in what they call a 'thermal comfort zone' we are all losing our brown fat and with it our capacity for thermoregulation. [1] And worse still, our nicely heated homes and offices are making our brown fat turn to white fat!

Ramp up fat burning through thermogenesis

The In-Sync Diet has focused on dietary and exercise recommendations to help you achieve your optimal body composition rather than optimal weight. By simply measuring your weight, you are not taking into account that you may be making huge improvements in your hydration levels and lean muscle tone to fat ratio. Indeed, the Body Mass Index (BMI) measurement, which is just a calculation using your height and weight, as an indicator of your health is not useful unless your body composition is taken into account.

Thermogenesis may be a handy tool to temporarily increase the rate at which you burn calories so that you lose fat and not lean tissue. This is a bit like stepping on the accelerator pedal and ramping up fuel consumption -

when thinking in terms of burning more calories, it is fantastic for achieving fat loss. This is separate from your Basal Metabolic Rate (BMR) which measures the amount of energy your body needs to stay alive. Your basal metabolism uses calories like a car engine that needs only a modicum of petrol to quietly tick over. And there are a number of ingredients that you probably often eat, if not every day that can activate your 'good' brown fat.

The In-Sync Diet list of thermogenic ingredients:

1. **Good quality animal protein** - eggs, fish, poultry and grass-fed meat.
    By ensuring that your diet is moderately high in quality protein, The In-Sync Diet has been promoting protein-induced thermogenesis. Protein cannot be stored in the body (unlike fat and carbohydrate) and so it stimulates brown adipose tissue to metabolise it quickly. This speeds up the rate at which you burn calories.[2]

2. **Black pepper**
    There is an extract in black pepper known as piperine that is thermogenic and also helps you to absorb nutrients from your food.[3]

3. Chilli peppers and sweet peppers

Chilli peppers and sweet peppers get their fiery heat from capsaicinoids. Capsaicinoids also promote thermogenesis and help you to burn calories.[4]

4. Green Tea

Green tea has a long history of use in supporting a healthy metabolism and body composition and can be considered a weight loss tool.[5]

5. Green Coffee Bean Extract

Green coffee bean extract is taken from green coffee beans that have not been roasted. They are a rich source catechins and caffeine and are used in supplements to promote weight loss.[6]

6. Turmeric

Turmeric is a spice associated with Indian cuisine. Curcumin is the yellow pigment that not only gives turmeric its colour, it also increases the rate of thermogenesis.[7]

Cold Water Therapy

Cold water therapy is just as the name suggests - immersing yourself in cold water to the point where you start to shiver. When you shiver, you use up calories to maintain your internal body temperature. It is a very useful therapy for the overweight and obese to bring the brown fat back.[8]

Before you plunge straight in, bear in mind that the immediate shock of the cold water could impact on your blood pressure! Start off by getting into a shower at your normal temperature. Then step out, turn the temperature to a cold setting and gradually acclimatise by sticking hands and feet and anything else you dare in until you are ready for the whole body experience. If you visit a spa and there is a cold plunge pool, this will have the same effect.

Glynis' Tip:

Well, I'm very pleased that all those days and nights spent filming outdoors in the middle of an English winter, over the years, did me some good! There were times when I was so cold I could barely speak, instead making barely intelligible sounds...and not even caring.

Being cold is my very worst thing! Not too keen on the

cold water thing I have to say but it's good when combined with jumping in and out of a sauna.

However, the thermogenic foods mentioned are big on my list of favourites. I switched to green tea many years ago and I have 1 or 2 cups every single day.

I love peppers and add them to my salad or vegetables on a daily basis.

Curcumin is a fantastic supplement in every way and I take it regularly. It's very good at helping deal with the inflammation that most people have going on in their bodies without even realising. Inflammation left unchecked leads to disease, health problems and premature ageing.

And, of course, it's completely thrilling to hear that a cappuccino is actually beneficial. The milk part not so much, but at least the odd cappuccino has some benefit. (Always better to combine with a meal rather than having on its own.)

Footnotes

1. Johnson F. et al. Could increased time spent in a thermal comfort zone contribute to population increases in obesity? *Obesity Reviews,* 12 543-551, 2011.
2. Westerterp K.R. Diet-induced thermogenesis. *Nutr Metab(Lond)* 1(1), 5, August 18[th,] 2004.

3. Badmaev, V, Majeed, M. et al. Piperine derived from black pepper increases the plasma levels of coenzyme Q10 following oral supplementation, The Journal of Nutritional Biochemistry.11 (2), 109-113, 2000.

4. Ludy M.-J., Moore G.E., Mattes R.D. The effects of capsaicin and capsiate on energy balance: Critical Review and Meta-Analyses of Studies in Human. *Chem Senses* 37: 103-121m 2012.

5. Belza A., Toubro S. and Ashrup A. The effect of caffeine, green tea and tyrosine on thermogenesis and energy intake Thermogenic effect of bioactive agents. *European Journal of Clinical Nutrition* 63, 57-64. Jan 2009.

6. Thom E The effect of chlorogenic acid enriched coffee on glucose absorption in healthy volunteers and its effect on body mass when used long-term in overweight and obese people. *J Int Med Res* 2007. Nov-Dec: 35 (6):900-8.

7. Manjunatha H. et al. Hypolipidemic acid and antioxidant effects of curcumin and capsaicin in high fed rats. *Canadian Journal of Physiology and Pharmacology,* Vol 85, No 6, June 2007.

8. Wilcock I.M. et al. Physiological Response to Water Immersion. *Sports Med,* 36(9) 747-765, 2006.

Chapter Sixteen

It is the everyday movements that count!

Challenging the culture of convenience

We live in a culture that aims to make life as convenient as possible. But is this really to our advantage or to our detriment? Researchers at the University of Missouri believe that our culture of convenience is contributing to the problem of obesity because it is removing the need to move around.[1] Fridges, water on tap, remotes for every electronic device, convenience food and internet shopping all deprive you from being able to make enough everyday movements that could potentially stop you from putting on weight ever! It is not only shivering that converts your white fat to 'good' brown fat to be burned for energy, everyday movements do this too. When you are active in your day to day lives you generate a newly discovered hormone in your muscles known as 'irisin' that is responsible for switching on genes that convert the white into brown.[2] Irisin is even capable of reprogramming your body's fat cells to burn energy rather than store it.[3]

Burn fat faster by intermittent natural movements through your day

You would not believe it but the short movements that you typically do through your day…

Stretching up to get something.

Reaching over to pick something up.

Bending down to do your shoe laces up.

Turning round to look back at something.

…can shift a load of calories and this is often more effective than a session in the gym or a cycle ride.

This accounts for why someone who is fidgety and cannot sit still is more likely to be slimmer than someone who may train every day but nevertheless has a sedentary job which means they spend a large part of their time sitting down.

Whenever you are up and about, the calories from your food are immediately converted into energy by your muscles to generate heat - thermogenesis. Everyday movements activate certain muscles that are known as the stabilisers of the body, the type II muscles that are associated with power sports and explosive bursts of activity.

Living in Gravity

Dr. Joan Vernikos, former director of NASA's life sciences division, believes the physical deterioration that happens to astronauts in space is similar to the ageing process on Earth as we become more and more sedentary - just the time scale is different. She says that by living sedentary lives we are not living 'in gravity' and that is contributing to a number of health problems including obesity.[4]

Living in gravity is all about regaining the energy and vitality you had as a child rather than spending your time sitting for hours. Sedentary behaviour is accompanied by physical changes in your body such as loss of muscle mass, increased fat mass, decreased bone density, floppy muscles, reduced explosive power and slower reaction time that is also felt by astronauts when they are suffering from Gravity Deprivation Syndrome. In her book 'Moving Heals Sitting Kills', Dr. Vernikos gives many ideas to help regain muscle tone and lose the fat.[4]

Some suggestions on how to add in everyday movements to 'live in gravity'

- Get into the stretching habit again especially whilst you are sitting at your desk or watching T.V. - this should include your arms and your legs.
- Bring flexibility to your joints by getting up from your desk and sitting down again (she recommends you do this at least thirty-five times per day).
- Change your posture every fifteen minutes of the day.
- Take a ride on a motorbike.
- Make use of balance plates at your gym.
- Stand tall - check your posture by leaning against a wall.
- Walk tall.
- Cook food from scratch.
- Dance.
- Play a musical instrument.
- Buy a balancing cushion to stand on.
- Do not always sit on a comfortable chair.
- Play a sport and get your children to play a sport too.
- Go out to shop rather than doing it online.

One study on a group of overweight seven to nine year olds revealed that all preferred to spend time playing with electronic games than going and doing sport.[5]

Top Tip:

In Chapter Seven The In-Sync Diet recommends measuring your movement with a pedometer to become more mindful of the amount of activity you do in a day. The generally accepted rule is that you should aim to be achieving up to 10,000 steps per day.

Glynis' Tip:

There's been much in the news of late about the dangers of prolonged sitting. I presumed I was absolutely fine with all my sitting because I exercise nearly daily. I was really shocked to learn that this is not the case. My lifestyle has changed dramatically in the last couple of years since I started my anti-ageing website. I now sit for many hours a day in front of my computer writing. It's very easy to lose track of time and quite often I find 4 or 5 hours have gone by.

I now make an effort to not sit for more than an hour (or less). I get up and go and make a cup of tea or just walk around the house doing some of my chores. A good idea if you're chained to a desk, is to set a timer for every 45 - 60 minutes. Go to the bathroom. Offer to get someone something they need. Take the stairs. Even just standing will help. Besides benefitting your general health, this will help keep the weight off. That's got to be a good motivation, hasn't it?

Footnotes

1. Hamilton M.T. Role of low energy expenditure and sitting in obesity, Metabolic Syndrome, Type 2 Diabetes, and Cardiovascular Disease. *American Diabetes Association*, Vol 56, No 11, pp 2655-2667, Nov 2007.
2. Courage K.H. Newly discovered hormone boosts effects of exercise and could help fend off diabetes. *Observations*. *Scientific American*. Jan 12, 2012
3. Vernikos J. 2011. Sitting Kills Moving Heals. Fresno, California, published by Quill Driver Books.
4. Bostrom P et al. A PGC1-1-dependent myokine that drives brown-fat-like development of white fat and thermogenesis. *Nature* 481, pp 463-480, 26th January 2012.
5. Carvalhal M.M. et al. Overweight and obesity-related activities in Portuguese children 7 - 9 years old. *The European Journal of Public Health,* Volume 17, Issue 1 pp 42-49. 22nd June 2006.

Chapter Seventeen

It's a wrap!

To be *In-Sync* means your body is responding to the changes we have recommended through the book and you are reaching your body composition goals. You have probably realised that The In-Sync Diet is not just another fad diet book, it is a diet and lifestyle book that is providing you with weight management tools, all backed by solid science, that you can employ for life. And of course managing your weight is not simply a question of eating less and exercising more although that helps!

So what are the fundamental aspects of The In-Sync Diet that you should keep with you to maintain a healthy body composition and a fantastic long life?

* **Water** - It is easy for us to assume that we are drinking enough because we are constantly drinking. But really we aren't and our cells are responding by storing fat. Rather than slipping back into old habits, aim to keep your water intake up by drinking plenty in one go and then not drinking again until you feel your thirst returning.

- **Avoid** the use of **artificial sweeteners** to get your sugary 'fix'. Your brain will expect calories that it simply is not getting and it will drive up appetite to make sure it does!
- **Move before you eat** - this is fundamental to maintaining a healthy body composition and good health for the rest of your life. When you move around on an empty stomach, your cells quickly adapt and become incredibly efficient at burning fat.
- All **exercise that you do on an empty stomach** will be beneficial. The In-Sync Diet has taken you from High-Intensity Interval Training, which is a great place to start if you have not exercised for a while, to how to introduce endurance exercise into your life.
- **Skipping breakfast** might be beneficial not only for your weight but your health also - by adopting a 'famine feast daily routine' you are activating longevity genes that will keep you alive and well for longer. You are also increasing your mitochondria to shift more fat.
- If you exercise in the evenings after work, it may be easier for you to eat breakfast, **skip lunch** and eat your second meal after your workout.
- Eat **two** (or three) **meals** per day. You are not genetically made for frequent eating and yet in modern life this is a situation that is hard to avoid. It is by leaving extended time between meals that you

will be changing from being a 'sugar burner' to a 'fat burner'.

- Eat a diet to reduce your lectin load. This means eating a diet that hardly includes **gluten grains** or **pulses**. You can at this stage add rice and gluten-free oats back into your diet if you wish. You will, on the whole, be eating a diet rich in quality protein and plant foods with plenty of healthy fat.

- Choose foods that support the health of your **mitochondria**. These are the powerhouses of your cells that provide the energy for your body - as their capability declines so does the capability of every organ and tissue in your body. By supporting them, you are also supporting your youthful vitality.

- Don't be too quick to turn on the heating in winter and enjoy cold showers in summer. By **shivering a little,** you are activating your brown fat which will help you to burn calories.

- Remember that **constant movement** through your day will stimulate a hormone, irisin, which converts white fat into brown fat to be turned into energy. A moderately high protein diet and **thermogenic compounds** such as chilli and turmeric will help this process too.

- Reduce your **over-response to stress** by employing techniques such as yoga and meditation each day that will allow you to remove yourself from issues that are bothering you so that when you look at them again, you can appreciate them in a new light. You will also have lots more energy!

- Be mindful of your **biological clock**. If you are an early bird and go to bed or eat just that little too late, you will feel it the next day and so will your body. If you happen to be a night owl, make sure you are getting your eight hours of sleep.

By being *In-Sync,* you are turning back the clock. Your chronological age is defined by the number of years you have been alive. There is no way of altering that! Your biological age, on the other hand, is related to the amount of wear and tear you have subjected your body to. Your biological age can be reduced by your good health and fitness.

Your biological age can actually be measured nowadays. It is done by looking at your telomeres that become frayed with age. Telomeres are the protective outer coatings on your DNA. By putting into practice all the strategies we have given you in **The In-Sync Diet** you are literally preventing your telomeres from becoming frayed and slowing down the ageing process.

Glynis' Tip:

You are now entering the trickiest part of this diet. The rest of your life.

How do you see the rest of your life? I like to see mine as healthy, active, engaged with everything around me and looking good. This desire has lead me to create my website and write this book.

In the couple of years I've been working with Fleur, I've made some fundamental changes to the way I eat and drink that I feel sure will be permanent. This is unusual for me because I've never stuck with a diet for longer than a few weeks in my life. However, the science behind this is very solid and the results have been undeniable, so there's no going back for me.

The basic changes are the guidelines that are mentioned above.

- *I no longer eat breakfast, but rather aim for 2 meals a day.*
- *I exercise in a fasted state.*
- *I don't snack.*
- *I drink plenty but only when thirsty and/or at certain times of the day.*
- *I avoid grains and gluten as much as possible*
- *I do eat a bit of dairy but not every day.*

However, this does not happen every single day. There are times when I wake up famished (usually after a drink the night before) and I have breakfast.

Sometimes my work schedule is very anti-social and I have to exercise at odd times or not at all (running around on stage is sometimes all the exercise I can handle). These odd working hours and not always having the kind of food I want available can make it very challenging at times. I do the best I can.

I try and stick to the basic rules above, making the mainstay of my diet, protein, vegetables and fruit with a small amount of natural unsalted nuts. It's the other things I add on top of this that can cause problems. Oh yes, I'm partial to my glass of rosé, my slice of cake (gluten free usually but at the end of the day, cake is cake), fries and desserts. Sometimes during a very social time or when I'm away, it all gets a little out of hand and I then put myself fully back onto the regime for a couple of weeks to get myself back on track. (I would recommend going to Phase Four, if you do this without the luxury meal.)

Doing the regime fully a few times a year is a great way to keep on the path of health and weight maintenance. You could do it for a week, 2 weeks (or longer if you're up for it), or even for a day after a few days of indulgence, whenever you feel the need or want to shift some weight. It's all up to you and whatever you want to achieve. The good thing is that after the 8 weeks you've just completed, you will be primed and conditioned to make these changes to your diet, that will, hopefully, become a way of life for you.

Congratulations for having taken on this challenge, for making these significant changes to your diet that will hugely impact your health, your longevity and energy levels.

For more lifestyle, health and beauty tips check out my website www.AgelessbyGlynisBarber.com

Exclusive Facebook Members Group

Now that you have your copy of The In-Sync Diet you can join the exclusive In-Sync Members group on Facebook! In the exclusive members group you will be able to have additional support from Fleur and Glynis and gain access to exclusive new recipes, meal ideas and additional hints and tips. Here you can also share your photographs of your success, stories and journey and even your menu ideas or recipes with your fellow In-Sync members.

To access the Facebook group visit www.InSyncDiet.com where you will be automatically redirected to the group or go to www.Facebook.com/groups/InSyncDiet/, then simply click 'Join group' and send a Facebook private message to, Fleur Borrelli, quoting 'VIP In-Sync'. Please do not share this access information with anyone else. This is an exclusive and safe private group for support and sharing with other members of The In-Sync Diet family.

Quotes on The In-Sync Diet from AgelessbyGlynisBarber.com

OMG! I'll never be as good as you but after a couple of comments from friends, I just jumped on scales & for the first time in almost 5 years it read 8 something instead of 9 something!!! Woohoo! & it's all thanks to you! (& the fact I have to get into a bikini this week!) Was always around 8st 4 'til my late 30's then it seemed suddenly, overnight I gained a body that wasn't mine & just blamed it on age! Don't weigh myself often as for me it's more about how I feel & how my clothes fit, plus I gain weight when I work out, but around 5 years ago I began keeping a record as I was creeping towards the dreaded 9 & a half st mark & seriously thought my 8st days were long gone! Now, how to keep going & keep it off... You're a great inspiration! Thank you

Amanda

Thank you again for the idea of the 'Boot camp'! I have lost 32 pounds since April and I feel so good! I love the way my husband looks at me again. It is great to see and feel men turning their heads. And last and not least, I am happy that I have made my son proud - he says he is proud that his classmates want me to be their teacher, because I am the prettiest teacher in our school :-). (Hope he will still be proud when he reaches his teens - he is 7 now.)

Blanka

I don't know whether you will remember me emailing you a couple of months ago at the start of my "Boot camp" to lose weight and tone up in time for a wedding last weekend? Well, I promised to let you know how I got on and despite a few hiccups along the way, I did it and I can honestly say I have never felt better. I now have so much more energy and my clothes fit me comfortably again! The first week was the hardest but once I got into it I found it quite easy. I don't particularly enjoy the gym so did lots of power-walking with the dog instead, as well as Yoga. I am now 9st 4lbs and will hopefully be able to maintain this reasonably easily. So thank you for all the advice and inspiring me to get back into shape.

Sarah

I turned 45 years old last month (and in the throes of the menopause) I really didn't like what I saw in the mirror. It was my tipping point. I sat down and went through the Ageless website with a fine tooth comb. I picked out bits here and there that would work for me and came up with a plan of action. I've dropped down from my size 16 and am nearly back to size 12 once again!! Thank you so much. Keep up the fabulous work with the website.

Elaine